box
INTO SHAPE

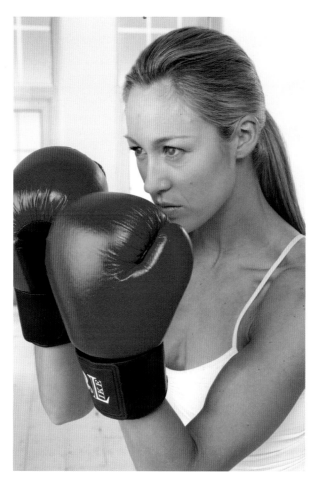

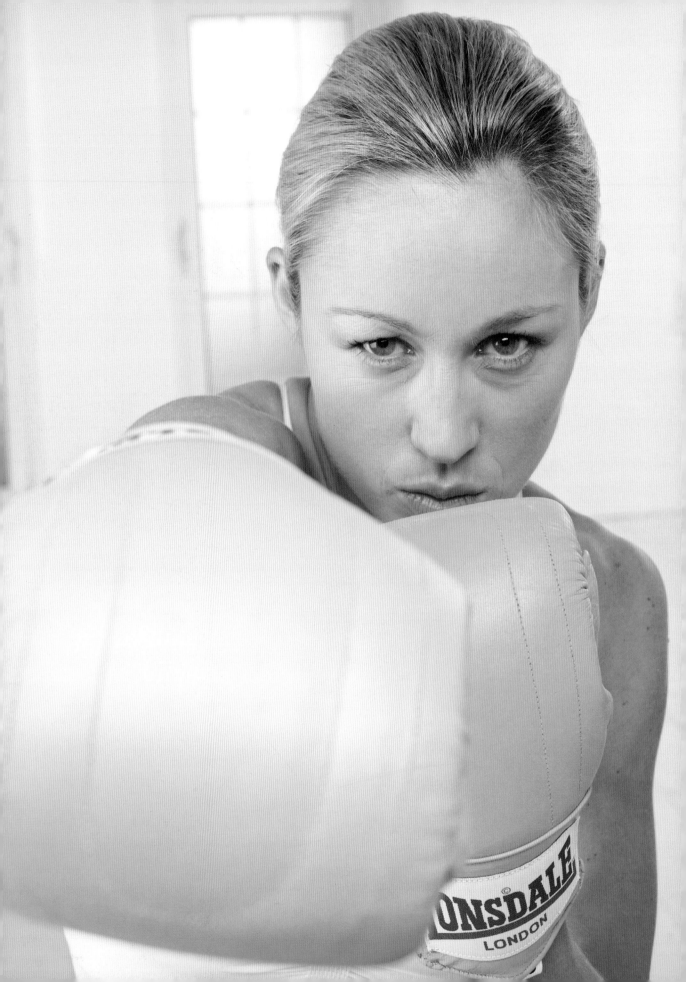

box
INTO SHAPE

Get fighting fit in just 12 weeks

Chrissie Gallagher-Mundy

hamlyn

For Tony, Killian & Finn — who are always fighting fit!

An Hachette Livre UK Company
www.hachettelivre.co.uk

First published in Great Britain in 2009 by
Hamlyn, a division of Octopus Publishing Group Ltd
2–4 Heron Quays, London E14 4JP
www.octopusbooks.co.uk

Copyright © Octopus Publishing Group Limited 2009

Distributed in the U.S. and Canada by Octopus Books USA:
c/o Hachette Book Group USA
237 Park Avenue
New York NY 10017

ISBN 978-0-600-61836-2

A CIP catalogue record for this book is available from the
British Library.

Printed and bound in China

10 9 8 7 6 5 4 3 2 1

Caution
It is advisable to check with your doctor before embarking
on any exercise programme. A doctor should be consulted
on all matters relating to health and any symptoms that may
require diagnosis or medical attention. While the advice and
information given in this book is believed to be accurate and
the instructions given have been devised to avoid strain,
neither the author nor the publisher can accept any legal
responsibility for any injury or damage sustained as a result
of following the advice in this book.

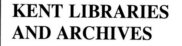

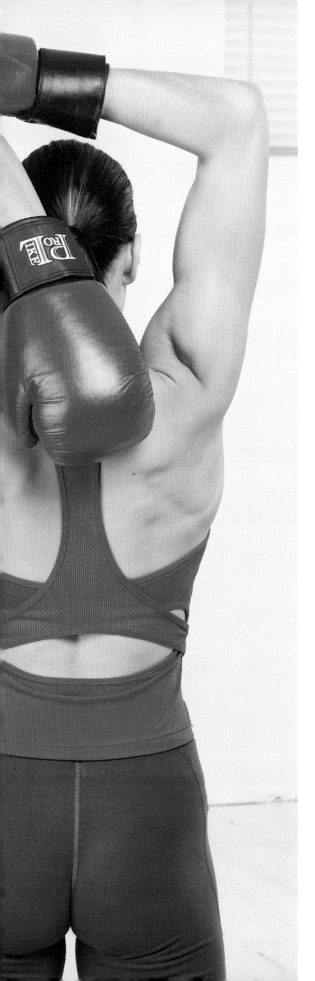

CONTENTS

INTRODUCTION

Getting fit via boxing is a new kind of workout – one where you focus your mind and your body to get your whole being fit, and have fun at the same time! It's a modern approach that derives from a long line of traditional sports and martial arts, and is now popular throughout the western world. Angelina Jolie and Jennifer Lopez both reportedly practise kick boxing and self-defence workouts.

MIXED TRADITIONS

Boxing workouts include a mix of techniques from the traditional boxing ring, such as the range of punches, and combines them with martial arts moves from taekwondo and karate, like the emphasis on stances and short, powerful movements such as blocks or strikes.

Martial arts are much more about defence than attack. On the other hand, boxing is essentially an aggressive pastime that developed as early as the third millennium BC. It was the Greeks who first started to formulate rules for the event so that eventually it became a 'sport'. By combining the aggression of boxing and the respect for defence of the martial artist you will learn the discipline of sharp, fast, controlled moves executed with thought and intent that builds power with purpose.

BOX YOURSELF FIT!

Over the years, fitness classes and styles have changed and evolved. While boxing has always been around as a hardcore sport, it has now permeated the gym and health club class to become a workout for all ages and levels of exerciser that really gets participants motivated and enthusiastic.

This book brings you all the different elements that can make up a boxing-style class. Throughout, you will experience the buzz and excitement involved when you get punching with your arms, kicking with your legs and twisting with your torso.

Specific health benefits from boxing fitness include increased muscle mass and improved co-ordination from the punches and conditioning work, better cardiovascular function from the jumps and kicks, and enhanced self-esteem from the focused approach of the workout. This truly is an all-round workout!

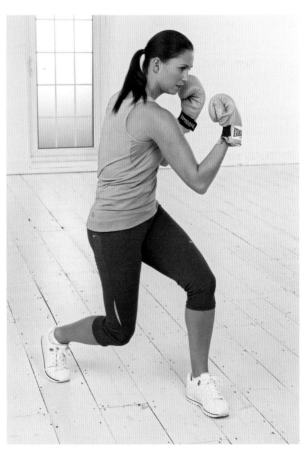

RELEASE YOUR INSTINCTS

Modern life can be stressful and a boxing workout can help to relieve your frustration by allowing you to hit out and explode – as your body was built to do – in a safe environment. One of the reasons boxing and martial arts are so popular is that they tap into our basic instinct to let off steam from time to time and express ourselves freely. All too often in everyday life we are constrained in what we can do, and spend our time concentrating on minutiae and avoiding conflict in social situations, which leaves no release for our natural 'fight or flight' mechanism.

Remember how you feel when someone says something that really upsets and annoys you? You want to hit out or run away, but of course you don't. The consequence is a release of adrenalin that is put to no good use and, over time, can cause harm to your body. So here is a great way to relieve tension, vent your anger and channel those feelings of frustration in a controlled and harmless way, and then put them to good use.

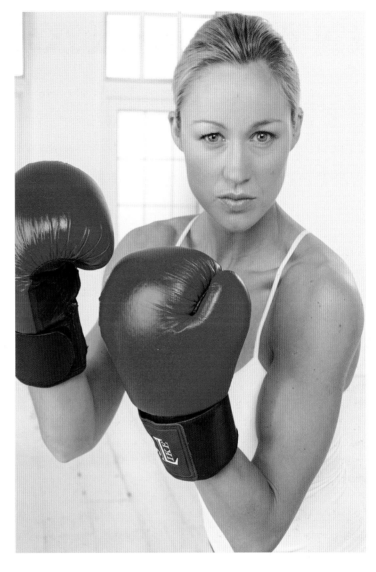

A POWERFUL WORKOUT

You can make use of your feelings – positive *and* negative – to fuel your exercise session, so that you are focused and investing your emotion and commitment into the moves to achieve the best workout ever. The more you concentrate, the better the results: if you exercise mindlessly and without a plan, your improvement tends to plateau and leave you feeling de-motivated. With boxing workouts there is a narrative, a 'story' that engages and focuses you, so that you move with intent and travel with energy. Your body then changes fast.

There are many elements to a boxing fitness workout and this book builds up your knowledge gradually, so that eventually you will have all the parts of the picture to put together. You can then use it to do a full workout at home at any time or as a back-up to any other form of exercise.

This book will allow you to take the first steps towards letting go. Discover the freedom of unleashing your pent-up energy and stress, having great fun – and getting fit in the process!

HOW TO USE this book

To get the most from this book, you need to use it regularly. Boxing fitness uses moves from the boxing, martial arts and fitness worlds, and some of the combinations and techniques require practice. The more you practise, the better you will become at them and the bigger the changes you will see in your body.

GET WITH THE PROGRAMME!

This programme is designed to make you feel and look better in just 12 weeks of regular working out. A suggested 12-week starter plan is provided in Chapter 5 'Fight Fit', along with a range of other routines designed to help you combine the moves you will have learned (see pages 92–123). You can use a variety of these to ring the changes and keep your workouts interesting. The Quick Workouts on pages 106–111 allow you to concentrate on particular areas that may need attention and ensure that you can exercise even if you are short of time. Alternatively, you can work straight through the chapter in order if you wish.

THE REGIME

Your boxing fitness sessions should follow the outline given below. Including each of these sections in your workout means you derive maximum benefit from the exercises.

Warm-up

Always start your workout with a basic warm-up (see pages 28–29). Do enough marching and toe downs to make you feel warm, then several dynamic stretches to prepare your muscles (see pages 30–31).

Next, move on to the skipping work on pages 46–47. This will begin to challenge your cardiovascular system, training your heart and lungs to be more efficient; it will also ensure you are thoroughly warm and, ideally, sweating – which indicates your warm-up has been sufficient – before you start working on techniques.

Conditioning

You should now move on to conditioning work. The exercises on pages 32–45 will help you build the basic strength you need to stay strong and aligned as you work

SAFETY FIRST

Before you begin and while you are still learning, it is best to read through each chapter in full first, taking careful note of any safety points as you go, before selecting a move or routine to practise. This will ensure you get the most from your workout without risking injury to your muscles and joints.

* Always warm up before starting your workout (see pages 28–31).

* Throughout, follow the instructions on stances and techniques exactly while you are learning, and then stick to them.

* Stay light on your feet and remember to pivot your toes to protect your knees.

* Keep your fists lifted with your arms protecting your body, and don't lock out your joints when punching (see pages 20–21).

* At any point, if you feel excessive strain or even pain, stop immediately.

* Always cool down at the end of your workout (see pages 48–51).

your technical moves. It is very important that your mid-section is supple and the abdominals are strong so that your back is protected. This will allow you to move with force but stay safe, at the same time flattening your stomach area to produce an improved appearance.

Technique practice

The next part of your workout should concentrate on specific moves from the boxing and martial arts repertoires. Choose one or two moves from Chapter 3 'Knock-out Body' and begin to work them. Work through the technical points and repeat the moves on both sides several times to get the correct feel and force. Then choose one or two moves from Chapter 4 'Kick-perfect Legs' and again work through the techniques and repetitions. Always include some balance work from this chapter, too.

Build your repertoire over 12 weeks (see pages 96–101), adding one new move at a time, and then start practising combinations. Add in the boxer's circuit and pyramids as alternatives at around week 4. By week 12 you will have learned all the moves and be in a position to perform a different combination of them in each workout.

Combinations

Once you've honed your technique, you can start to put some of your moves together. In the beginning, when you haven't yet learned the complete repertoire of moves, you can combine just the few you have learned. Use some of the agility moves on pages 76–77 and 102–105, and try to move around your space as you throw in a jab or hook or front kick – whatever new move you may have mastered. Keep the movement going, bouncing and jogging as you build up to your next move, and then put that into the mix. Work on all this for 10 minutes or so.

As you advance and learn more upper and lower body moves, you can then work through some of the combinations suggested in Chapter 5 'Fight Fit'.

Cool-down

It is essential that you always cool down after your session with the stretch and rub-down routines provided on pages 48–51. Stopping suddenly after an intense workout session is not good for the body. Stretching and cooling down gradually allows your circulation to slow gradually and your muscles to return to their pre-workout length. It also gives your mind some much-needed time for relaxation.

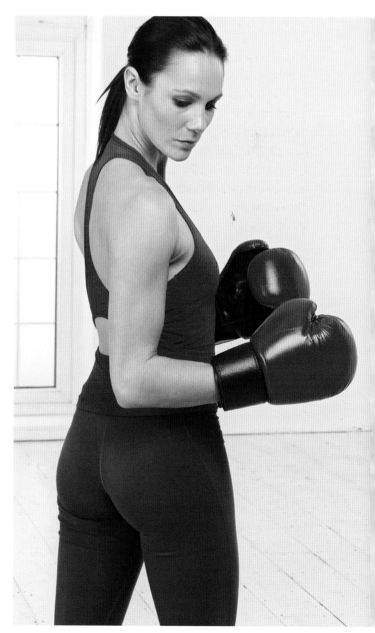

LEVELLING UP

In this kind of workout there are no beginner or advanced moves: each move needs to be technically correct from the start and should be approached in that way. However, you can increase the level of difficulty as you improve and become more familiar with a particular technique. Below are some general guidelines; specific instructions are provided for individual exercises where appropriate.

Level 1

Start by performing the moves slowly. Think about the technique points provided and work through these as you perform the move. Check your foot position, core engagement (see page 32) and alignment.

Level 2

Keeping all the above in mind, now start to focus on your intention. Focus on your phantom opponent and perform each move with increased energy and strength. Get into the story and start to think aggressively, move stealthily, and hit and kick with commitment. This will fire more muscles, use more energy and ultimately hone your body more quickly.

Level 3

Use all the commitment from Levels 1 and 2 and now travel the moves. Move all around the space you have available and use every corner. Study the agility moves on pages 76–77 and 102–105 and use the techniques to take you every which way as you perform some devastating kicks and punches!

MUSIC

Music is a great motivator and can be an important part of your workout. Use it to fuel your aggression, raise your energy and give impetus to your moves. Seek out high-energy music and make a playlist of your favourite uplifting tracks that will really inspire you, then use the music to help you punctuate and accentuate different moves. After your technique work, if your living arrangements allow, turn up the volume for the combos and really GO FOR IT!

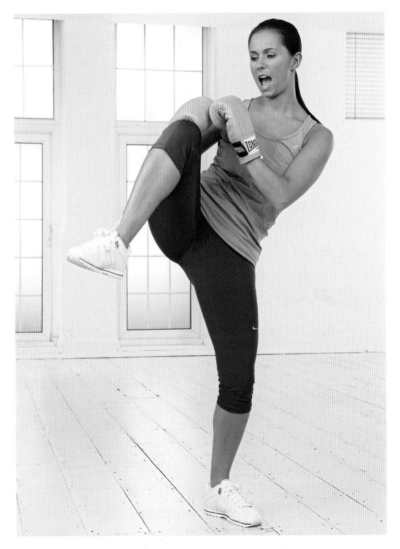

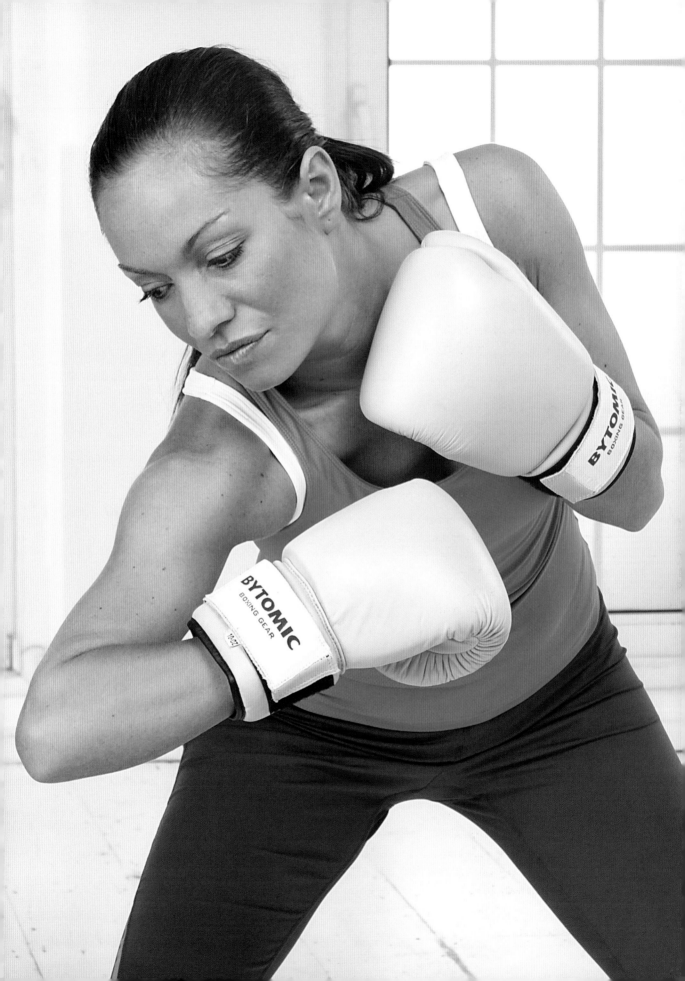

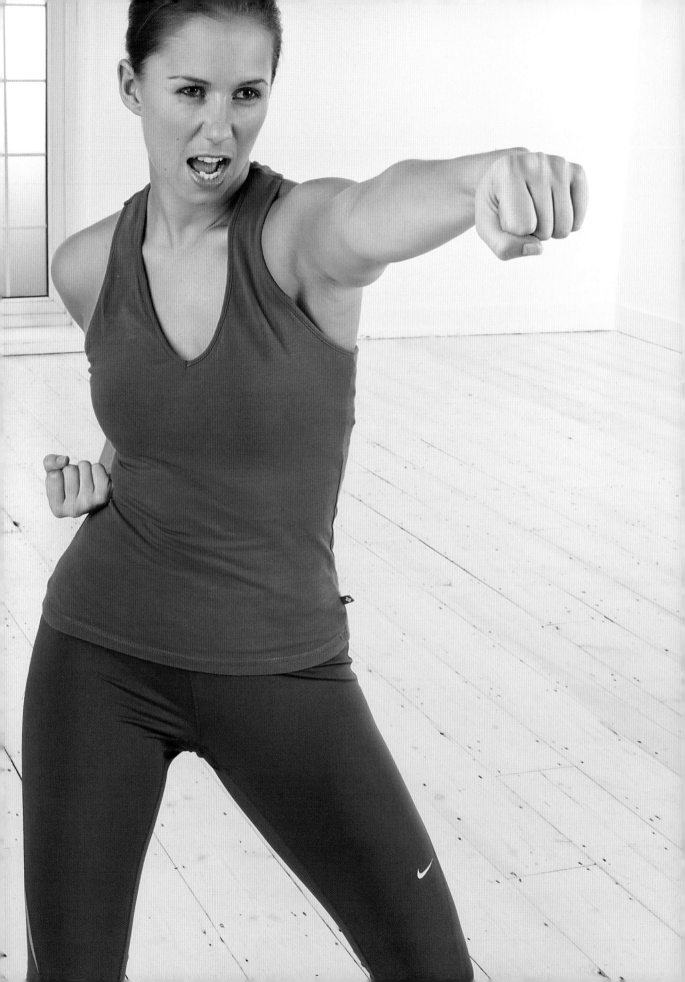

THE BOXING DIFFERENCE

In this chapter you will learn first about how to organize your home workouts, then about the types of session you may come across if you attend boxing or kick-boxing sessions at a gym. Don't forget that you can always go to classes at the same time as working with this book. You will then be introduced to the importance of the boxer's mindset, and the basic principles of attack and defence. This is the start of a new you!

best PRACTICE

This book will help to give you a taste of the boxing workout experience by learning the basic moves and 'feels' to get you started. Once your training progresses, you may decide to join a class at the gym or attend one of the many public training sessions offered at boxing establishments.

HOME WORKOUT

One of the best ways to get fit is to have a workout routine that you can do in your own home. This way, if you cannot get to the gym or have missed your class, you can still keep up your practice so you won't feel you have missed out.

Make a commitment

Practice is the key to all fitness and to you achieving your boxing best, so start making some time in your schedule now. In order to improve at anything you need to practise it at least three times a week, so aim for this frequency of training in order to progress quickly when you start.

Space to move!

On pages 16–17 you will find descriptions of a variety of equipment that can enhance your training, but you don't need much at all to get started. For the boxing workouts described in this book you will be using techniques from traditional boxing, kick boxing and martial arts, which can all be performed with a minimum of equipment. However, you do need to check your workout space.

First and foremost, a space for training must be free from clutter. You can use any room, a garage or your garden as long as there are no overhanging or protruding objects. Remember that you will be extending your arms and legs in all directions and that some moves require you to move around, so walk about in your space swinging your arms and kicking your legs out wide to check for any potential hazard.

If you can place a large mirror in the space, this will help you hone your technique and it will provide a focus for shadow boxing by checking your posture and shape.

Finally, make sure that the room is well ventilated. You will be punching and kicking up a sweat so make sure you can throw open a window and let in some fresh air.

TAKE NOTE

* The techniques described in this book are for non-contact and non-combat situations. They are NOT intended as self-defence or fight strategies.

* This book is NOT a self-defence manual – it is written for those who want to have fun while exercising and working on fitness.

* The techniques described here are not a substitute for professional boxing or kick boxing training. They are intended primarily for exercise at home *without* a sparring partner.

* Should you wish to become a real boxer and fight with contact, approach your local boxing gym for advice on how you might begin that type of training.

JOIN THE CLUB

If you want to further your practice by attending a boxing class, numerous options are available. Health clubs often offer boxing-style sessions that might include a body combat class, shadow boxing, or work on kicking bags and pads. There are also classes that involve the use of equipment such as focus pads and boxing gloves. These sessions will be led by health professionals who have learned how to incorporate boxing-style conditioning into their routines so the class should be well structured.

Another type of regime is available to you through the many boxing gyms that exist for professional and amateur fighters. These gyms contain the traditional boxing ring along with most of the equipment used to train a professional

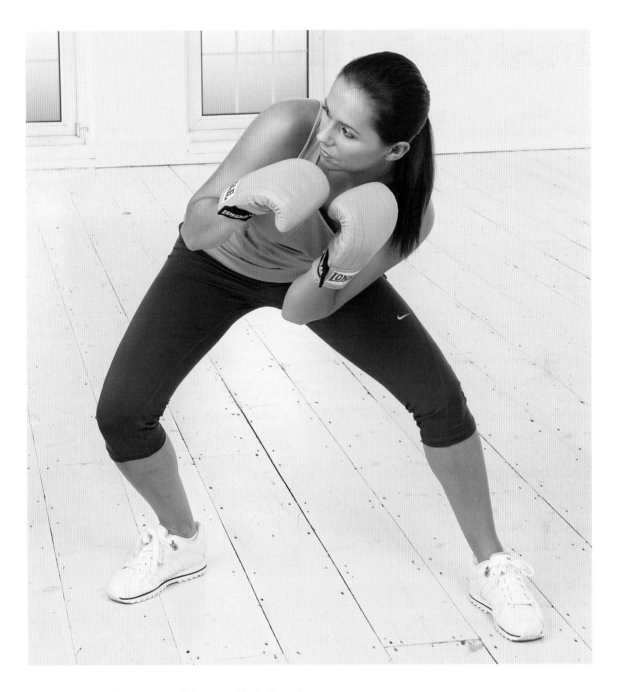

fighter. This kind of atmosphere will be more akin to the real boxing experience and focuses on techniques specific to that sport, so it is usually more popular with men. However, there may be less emphasis on modern gym safety standards. You will be training at your own risk, so always check out the place carefully and make sure your instructor has modern qualifications that allow him or her to teach safely. Always perform a warm-up and cool-down, and allow yourself a rest day between sessions.

EQUIPMENT

The equipment described here is used by professional boxers for safety and training purposes. For your workout, only the skipping rope is essential, but you might want to experiment with focus pads and bags at the gym.

AT HOME

There is only one essential piece of equipment you will need in order to get started on your home workout. The rest are optional – although a mirror is extremely useful – and guidance as to their suitability for use at home is given under their individual descriptions.

Skipping rope

This is great for improving your stamina, agility and footwork. It is also an excellent warm-up tool.

Mirror

When working at home, you can use a mirror instead of a sparring partner to aid posture and focus – but make sure you stand well back to avoid any possibility of smashing it!

AT THE GYM

If you attend a boxing fitness class at a gym or health club, you will probably use one or more of the following items of equipment at some point.

Focus pads

These are pads that usually have target spots on them and are worn by a partner for the boxer to hit. You may well work with focus mitts in pairs at a class.

Bags

Many different types of bag are used for hitting practice. A bag allows the boxer to work on target practice, hand–eye co-ordination and speed, as well as practising combinations. Freestanding versions filled with sand or water for stability can be used at home if you have the space. Bags that hang from a chain, whether large or small, are best confined to a professional gym.

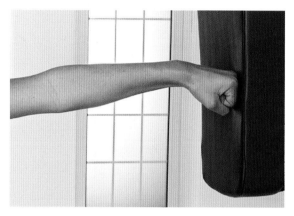

Focus pads can improve your technique.

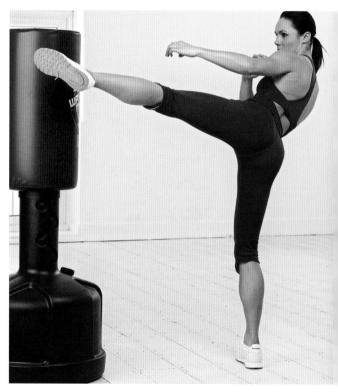

Freestanding bags are good for target practice.

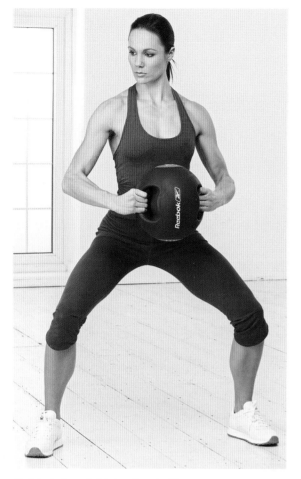

Medicine balls can build strength and agility.

Mouth guard

A mouthpiece or gumshield is always worn by boxers (and also by rugby players) to protect the inner mouth and lips from being cut if the boxer receives a hard blow to the face. The shield also helps to lock the top and bottom jaws together, to minimize damage to the jaw joint capsule if a boxer is landed by a hook. You will be learning hooks – but not on someone's jaw! A mouth guard is required only if you are sparring with a partner.

Gloves

There are many different types of glove available, ranging from light designs used when practising the speedball (see pages 62–63 for the shadow version) to heavier gloves for sparring or hitting heavy bags. Gloves protect the knuckles and reduce the risk of hand injuries during hitting practice. Sparring gloves are used in real fights, so are essential in practice for professional boxers.

Medicine ball

This weighted ball is used to practise handling speed and weight, often when working with a partner in a box-fit class. It is available in a range of weights.

Hand wraps

Hand wraps are sometimes used for boxing workouts, to protect the fingers and knuckles. They are not essential, and gloves are preferable when you are actually hitting something.

Headgear

Headgear is used to protect the boxer's head against soft-tissue damage such as bruises and cuts. A feature of amateur but not professional boxing, headgear does not protect against stuns and blows, so the boxer must always be on the defence to avoid such contact. It is only necessary if you are sparring with a partner.

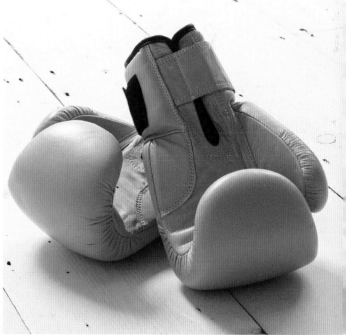

Gloves protect the whole hand when punching.

mind GAMES

The great thing about a boxing fitness session is that it's not like any other workout. You don't just turn up and run routinely through the moves. When you approach a boxing session you need to be focused and get into the story ...

MAKE IT REAL

You are a boxer or martial artist in the ring, facing a tough opponent. Each time you get up to train, that is the situation. This means committing to each move, and moving with conviction and intent. You must be focused and

MIND OVER MATTER

Even though you are not actually fighting a real person, it is important always to imagine your opponent opposite you – this will get your adrenalin pumping!

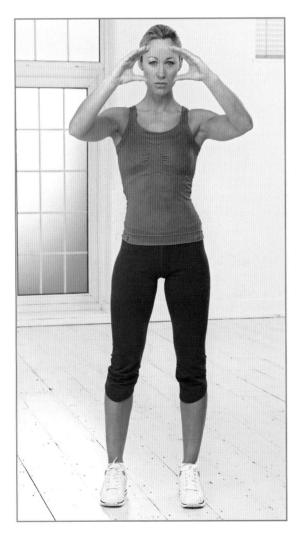

concentrating, thinking only about the quality and intensity of your moves and nothing else.

It also means concentrating from the moment you begin your warm-up, so that you are preparing both your body and your mind for the task ahead.

FOCUS YOUR WILL

Before you begin your workout each time, try some of these centring exercises to get you energized and focused.

Window focus

Stand with your feet hip width apart and shoulders pulled back and down. Bend your knees slightly and tighten your abdominals. Now lift your arms and form a window with your hands. Look through this window and focus at a point directly ahead. Do not allow anything to distract you from looking at that particular point.

Breathe in through your nose and out through your mouth, filling your lungs with air. Tighten the lower (transverse) abdominals to support your breathing. Take 5 long breaths as you focus your gaze and prepare your mind. Think about the workout (fight) ahead, and how you will commit to it and make your body work effectively and strongly.

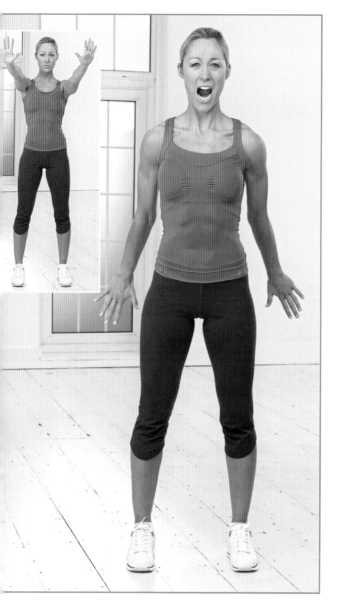

Get fired up

Stand with your feet hip width apart and knees slightly bent. Breathe in slowly through your nose while raising your arms in front of you, as far as your breath will take them. Spread your fingers and stretch out your hands. Now exhale forcefully and explosively through your mouth with a yelling sound, pulling your arms down as fast as you can. Repeat 3 times.

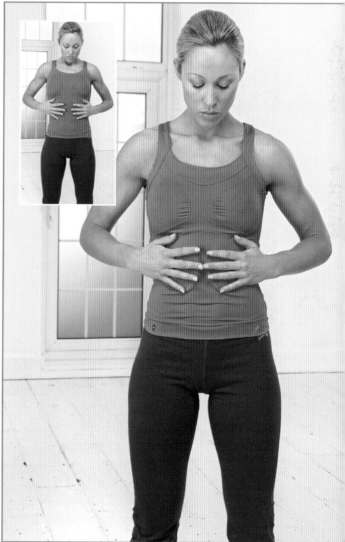

Breath of life

Breathing well is vitally important for all exercise – and for life! – so make sure you really use your ribcage and lungs to get the best possible inhalation. Stand with your fingers just touching, wrapped around your ribcage. As you inhale, notice how your fingers are pulled apart as your lungs expand and fill with air. Now exhale strongly, using your abdominal muscles to help, and notice how your fingers push back towards each other as your ribcage flattens again.

boxing basics:
DEFENCE AND ATTACK

To get the most out of your workout time, you need to be very clear about everything you are doing. As well as the basic boxing moves you will be mastering, you also need to learn transition moves and the correct positions to take in between sequences. Working through the core positions described in the rest of this chapter will ensure you are using all the right muscles and achieving the correct posture and attitude for this excellent kick-ass routine.

DEFEND YOURSELF

Whenever you are working on boxing fitness, you need to keep your guard up. This means thinking like a fighter and always protecting your body and head with your arms and hands raised.

Boxer's guard

Lift your arms and keep your fists tight, with your thumb over the top of your fingers. This will protect your thumb against

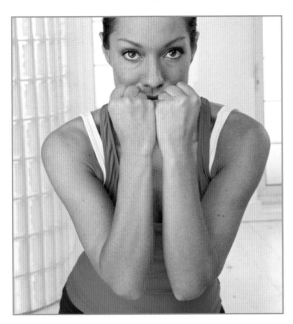

Keep your guard up to protect yourself.

getting broken, and once you have a glove on you can't get your thumb underneath. Keep your wrists straight and strong, with your fists at your jawline to protect your face. Your elbows should remain close to your ribs.

ON THE ATTACK

In your home workout, all your boxing moves will be shadow boxing and you won't be making contact with anything, unlike in a class where you may have the chance to kick or punch at a pad. You can still keep the aggression and energy in the moves – you'll just be saving on impact.

Fist technique

Despite the fact that you won't be hitting anything solid, you still need to make sure your hand is fisted correctly. Lift your hand palm up, curl your fingers into your palm and fasten your thumb over the top of your fingers. Turn your fist over and extend your arm out in front of you, looking down the line of your second knuckle. This is the fist you use for all your punches, sometimes turning it vertically.

Strike surface

The strike surface is the part of your fist with which you hit your opponent. If you were actually making contact with an aggressor you would aim to do so with the first two knuckles. You would never hit with the middle knuckles, otherwise you would break your hand! So, always aim your hand as if you will strike with the top of it.

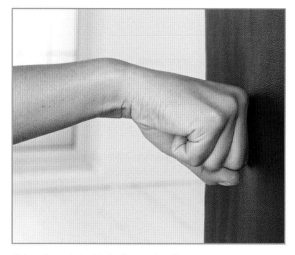

Only make contact with the first two knuckles

Agility

Besides thinking about hitting on target, you also need to concentrate on staying light on your feet. This might seem a contradiction when you're getting down low and using your body weight to throw punches, but good boxers and martial artists are also quick and agile on their feet.

Practise bouncing from foot to foot while keeping your guard up. You should be bouncing on your toes with your heels not far off the ground. Practise bouncing from side to side and forward to back in this way, so that you get used to moving like this the whole time. Boxers never stay still.

No straight slamming

In order to protect your joints when shadow boxing, it is very important that your moves are not too percussive. This means you should never slam your arms or legs straight.

For example, when you punch forward imagine your arm is on a piece of elastic, so that it springs back to your body after you have punched. Keep the move light and dynamic, but do not lock the joint as this could cause injury to your elbow. When you punch your imaginary partner, always keep your elbow bent just a little. You can still be aggressive and speedy while protecting your joints. Imagine a point in space where you are aiming to punch (see below), then punch through rather than at it so that the movement is strong and doesn't suddenly stop dead.

Punching (and kicking) in this way will allow you to use lots of energy and aggression but at the same time keep your joints safe.

Target zones

When you are punching, think about where you would actually strike a real opponent and then take aim. Don't punch wildly: if you were in a real fight, this would be disastrous. Each punch must be aimed at a specific area of your opponent's body. Target zones include the nose, chin, chest, stomach and groin. Imagine your opponent in every detail – particularly their height and weight – as you aim for these areas. Don't think aggression, think precision. That way you'll hone your techique to perfection!

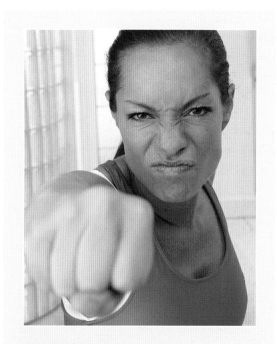

KEEP IN MIND
Don't forget the mindset of the boxer/martial artist:

* Action

* Aggression/spirit

* Discipline

* Commitment/perseverance

boxing basics: STANCES

In boxing fitness, how you stand is very important and is different to the stance used for a Pilates or toning class. The basic stance is with your legs hip width or 1½ times hip width apart (depending on the move you are performing) and your knees bent so that you feel low to the floor or grounded. Your arms should be up near your face in guard (see page 20) and your abdominals engaged (see page 32), forming a strong mid-section that is ready for movement or impact from your opponent.

STAND AND DELIVER

Two basic stances are used for the moves in this book: forward and combat. Combat stance is the stance most often used in real boxing matches. From here the boxer is protecting their upper body but able to deliver lightning thrusts with the arms at the same time. Forward stance is useful for travelling moves.

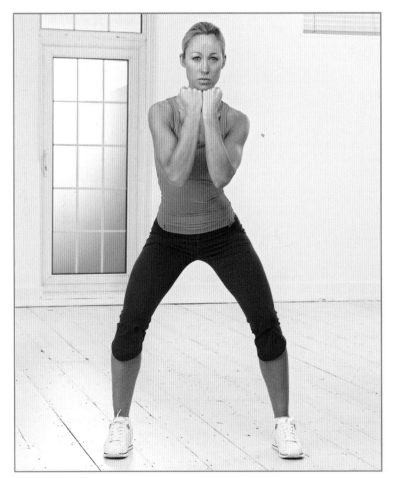

Forward stance

You will often begin a sideways-moving sequence from here. In a forward stance your whole body faces the front, with your eyes focused ahead and chin tucked in. Centre your weight between your feet, which should be 1½ hip widths apart and facing forward. Engage your abdominals and bend your legs slightly so that you are low and stable. Imagine that a threatening opponent is directly in front of you. This position looks and feels defensive yet ready for action!

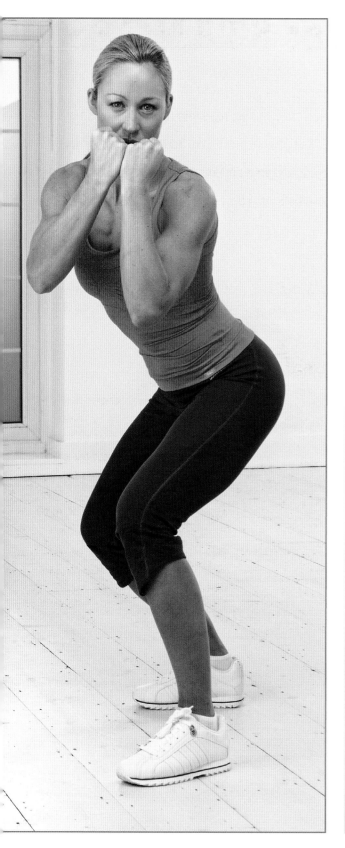

Combat stance

This is the stance from which you will aim your devastating punches! Face your opponent sideways on, with your feet hip width apart and arms up in guard. Your back foot should turn out at approximately 45 degrees. Position your fists at cheek height with your punching arm forward. Your body weight should be centred between your feet, but with the feeling that you could quickly transfer it from the back foot to the front as you punch. Check that your core muscles are engaged (see page 32) and your knees slightly bent.

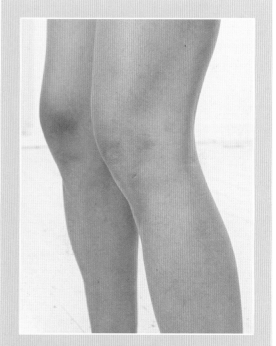

SAFE STANCE

Keeping your knees slightly bent avoids damaging impact to your knee joints and maintains stability and control for fast movement.

kick START

In Chapter 4 'Kick-perfect Legs' you will be learning a variety of kicks derived from martial arts moves that you can then incorporate into your boxing workout. In order to perform these moves without risk of injury to your muscles and joints, you need to keep a number of safety points in mind whenever you practise.

ALWAYS WARM UP

You should *always* warm up your whole body (see pages 28–31) before practising any technical parts of your workout, and this includes kicking. Going into a kick cold could result in a painful pulled muscle or tendon, and the end of your workout routine for some time.

In addition, practise a kick slowly before you perform it at full speed, to make sure the relevant muscles really are warmed up.

UNDERSTAND POSITIONING

Before you kick out, you will use the chamber position (see pages 78–79). Here the knee is drawn up close to your body, ready to be extended with force. This is the safe way to initiate a kick.

For a side kick, you need to tilt your hips in order to be able to extend your leg sideways easily (see pages 80–81). You will be aiming and making contact with your heel, so this is the part of the foot on which you should focus for the side kick, ideally keeping your toes lower than your heel.

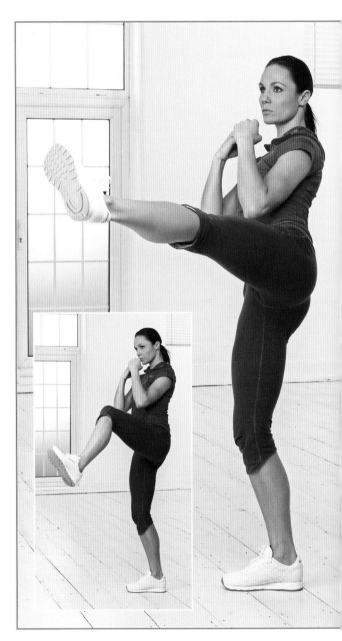

PIVOT TO PUNCH – OR KICK

When you throw a punch or perform a turning kick, you should lift your heel and pivot on the ball of your foot as your turn back and forth (for example, see pages 56–57 and 82–83). This will help you avoid any risk of twisting the knee or pulling joints or ligaments through excessive twisting.

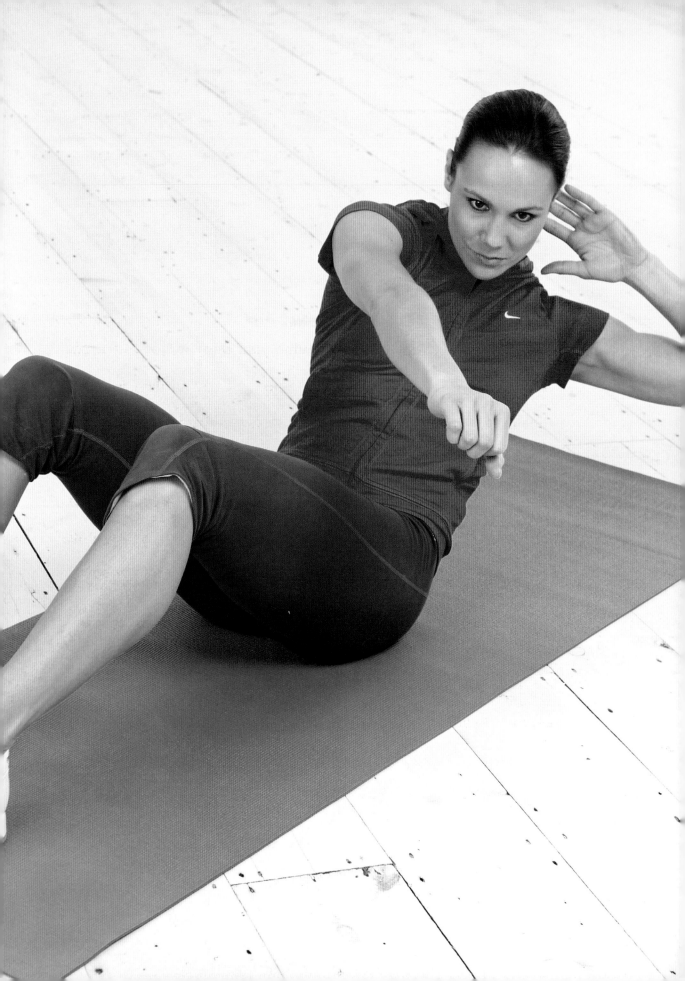

GET IN SHAPE

This chapter is all about conditioning your body to become extra muscular and toned. Being strong and properly aligned is a key tool in the boxer's arsenal, so you need to make time in your workout specifically for one or two exercises that address these areas. Building strength in key areas will allow you to perform the moves safely and more effectively. Keeping these areas strong throughout your life will also help you to maintain good posture, look taller and even avoid injury. The exercises in this section aim to challenge your muscles and put them under stress, so that they develop and strengthen. They can also be performed as a separate workout.

get MOVING

Warming up should be a part of any workout and boxing fitness is no exception. Before you start hitting, kicking and punching, your body as well as your mind should be prepared. Make the first 5–10 minutes a limbering and mobilizing section to warm up your body and prevent muscle damage or tendon strain when you start your workout. As well as the warm-ups described here, you may want to try the traditional boxer's conditioning exercises of jogging and skipping (see pages 43 and 46–47).

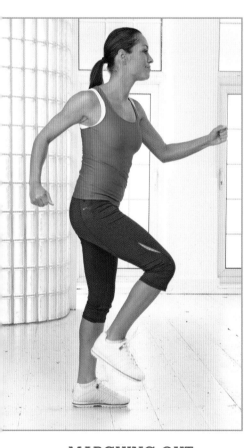

MARCHING OUT

Get your body moving and start to become light on your feet by marching on the spot. Lift your knees high and swing your arms vigorously to create some heat. Keep this up for 1 minute.

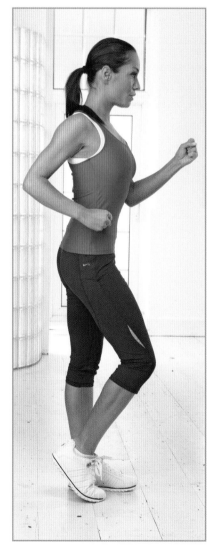

TOE DOWN

1 Now warm up your ankles and feet, as you'll be doing a lot of fast moves on them. Stand with your weight evenly distributed on both feet and lift up on to tiptoe as high as you can, then lower your heels back down with control. Repeat 4–5 times.

2 Now alternate the heel up, so that you are pressing down first one heel and then the other in a rhythmical motion. Repeat 4–5 times.

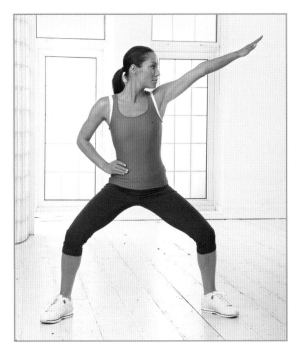

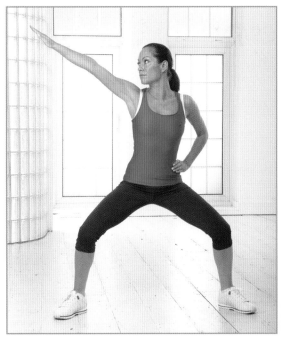

HALF STARS

1 Stand with your feet together and then step out to one side and bend your knees into a plié, throwing your arm out to the side.

2 Now bounce the same foot back in and step out to the other side. Repeat 10–15 times.

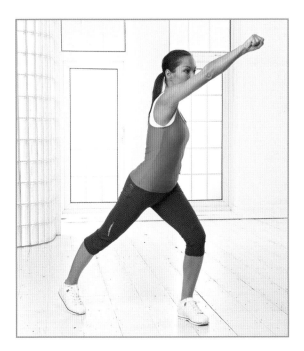

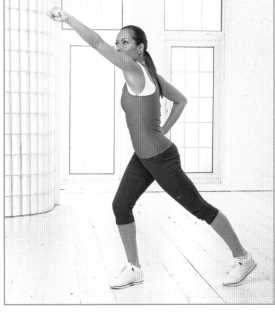

LUNGES

1 Start with your feet together, then step your right leg out to the side and slightly behind as you swing your right arm up.

2 Step your left leg out to the side and slightly behind as you swing your left arm up. Alternate left and right 10–15 times.

limber UP

Dynamic stretches are very useful warm-up tools for the boxer/martial artist as they allow you to stretch and prepare your body while moving and staying warm. At this stage, passive stretches would cool down your body too much. Performing the following stretches at speed will keep you warming up, and ready your mind and body for the dynamic moves to come. The boxing workout includes leg and arm work, so you need to prepare these body parts for what lies ahead.

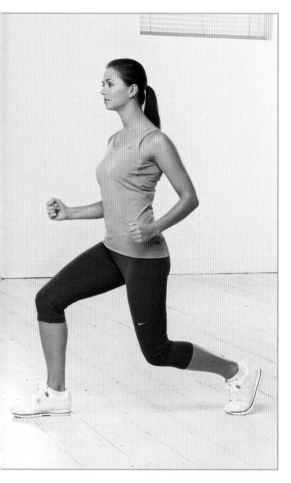
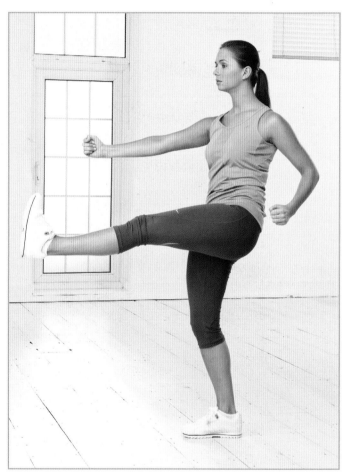

DYNAMIC HAMSTRING STRETCH

1 Stand in a lunge position with one leg behind you, heel raised. Your front foot should be flat and both knees slightly bent. Feet are parallel and facing forward.

2 Now push off your back foot to kick out the leg in front of you. As you bring your leg forward, bend the knee and then kick purposefully forward – you don't need to kick high. You will feel the stretch in your hamstring (back of the upper thigh) as you straighten your leg. Repeat 3 times on each side. As you loosen up you can start to kick higher to stretch a little further.

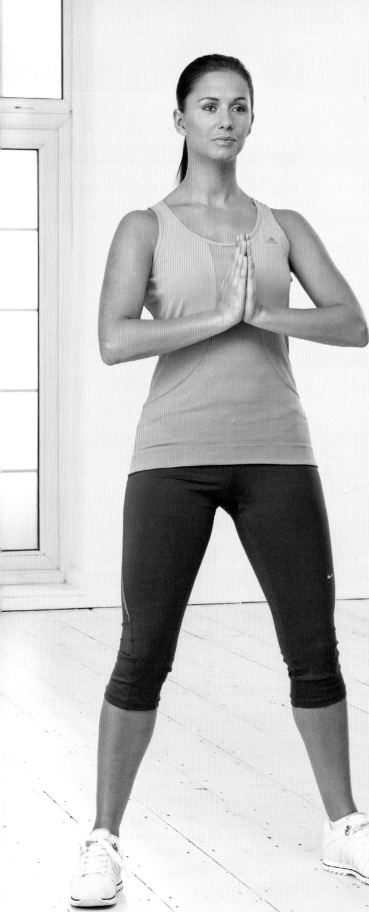

DYNAMIC CHEST STRETCH

1 To stretch your arms and chest, stand with your feet hip width apart and press your palms together.

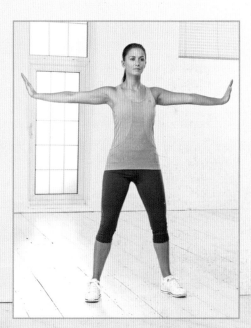

2 Now push your palms off each other as you extend your arms dynamically out to the side. Repeat this 3–4 times, then push your arms a little behind you as you extend them, so that you feel the stretch across your chest and biceps (front of the upper arm). Repeat 3–4 times.

Complete your warm-up with some skipping (see pages 46–47).

focus on: ABDOMINALS

One of the first areas of your body you need to get in shape is your mid-section. Your torso is the area that allows you to twist, lean and bend, while the muscles in this area also protect and support your spine. The stronger your mid-section, the flatter your stomach and the safer your back will be – so start strengthening now.

LEVELS

Level 1 Perform 5 reps.
Level 2 Add another 5 reps each time you train.
Level 3 Perform 50 reps.

GET ENGAGED

1 Lie on your back with your knees bent and feet flat on the floor. Place your fingertips just inside your hip bones and cough: you will feel your TVA contract. Keeping your fingers in position, breathe in, then breathe out as you pull your navel in towards your spine. Hold for a moment: you have now contracted your TVA. Release the muscles so that you can feel the difference, then tighten again. This should feel as if you are putting on a belt: pull the belt as tight as you can (contract your abdominals tightly), then let the belt out a couple of notches (release the contraction on your abdominals slightly, to about 30 per cent of your maximum contraction). Your TVA is now engaged – contracted for support, but not over-tightened – now your muscles are ready to support anything your torso wants to do. Repeat this in different positions (for example, standing upright), so that you become accustomed to the feeling of drawing in your stomach area in this controlled way. Also practise this posture at other times of the day when you are not exercising, so it becomes routine.

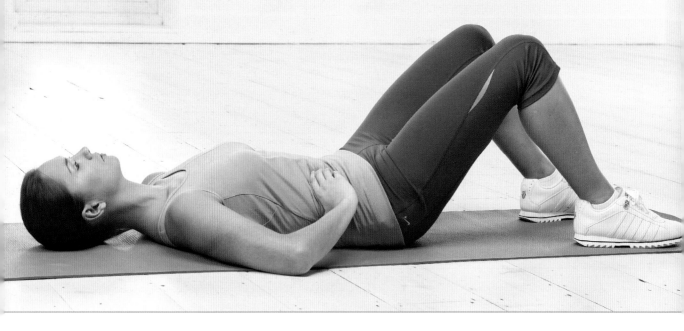

KNOW YOUR ANATOMY

One of the first conditioning techniques you need to learn is how to find and activate your transverse abdominal (TVA) muscles. These are the muscles that wrap horizontally around your abdomen and lie deeper than the rectus abdominis that normally shows on a bare stomach. They are very important muscles as they connect to both the rectus abdominis (the six pack) and the back muscles, and help to provide a stable corset around your middle.

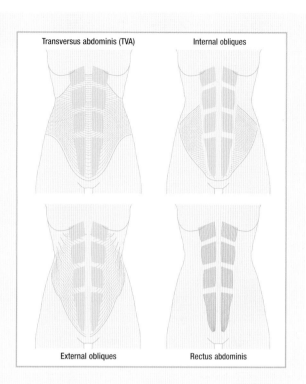

Transversus abdominis (TVA)

Internal obliques

External obliques

Rectus abdominis

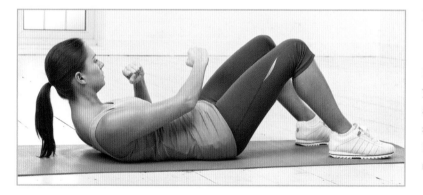

PUNCHING ABS

1 Lie on your back with your knees bent, press your lower back towards the floor and engage your TVA. Now contract your abdominals to lift your head, shoulders and ribcage off the floor in a curve, as you punch forward and up with your arms.

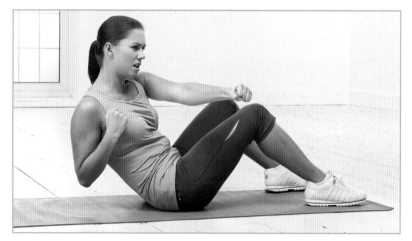

2 As you lift to the top of the curve, punch right and left with each fist across your body to knock out that opponent! Lower yourself back down and repeat.

ABS CYCLING

LEVELS

Level 1 Perform 10 reps.

Level 2 Add 10 reps of the variation.

Level 3 Add another 5 reps each time you train, building up to 40 in all.

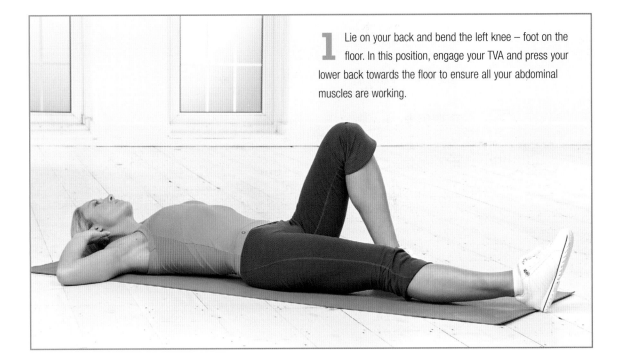

1 Lie on your back and bend the left knee – foot on the floor. In this position, engage your TVA and press your lower back towards the floor to ensure all your abdominal muscles are working.

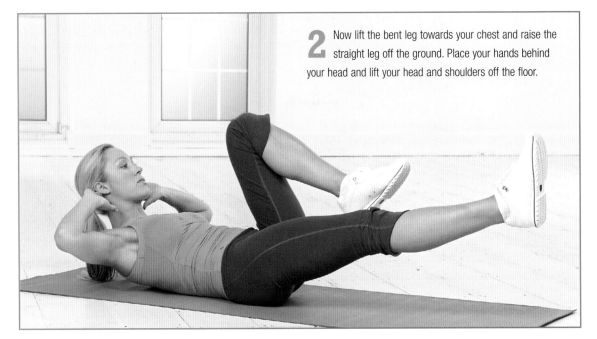

2 Now lift the bent leg towards your chest and raise the straight leg off the ground. Place your hands behind your head and lift your head and shoulders off the floor.

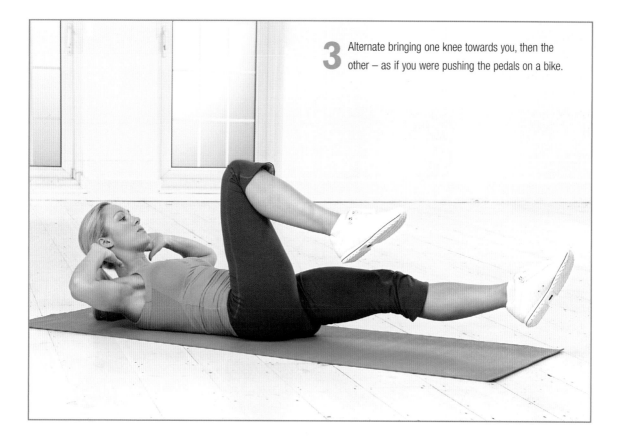

3 Alternate bringing one knee towards you, then the other – as if you were pushing the pedals on a bike.

VARIATION: TWIST

Try to touch your elbow to the opposite knee, so that your upper body is twisting as you move each leg and you are looking to the side as your upper body turns.

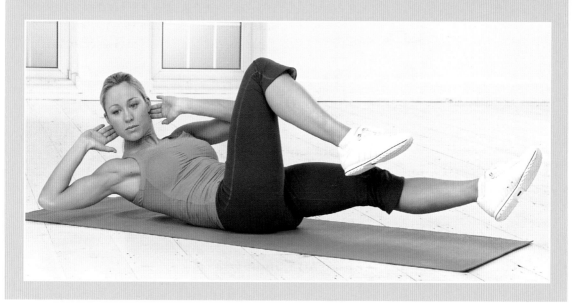

focus on: BACK MUSCLES

It is important to keep your back muscles as strong and as supple as you can. Because these muscles contribute less to appearance than to alignment they are often overlooked, but good posture is important and will help make you look more youthful. As well as strengthening the muscles, you should also keep your back as supple as you can, and this means moving it in all directions. In everyday life you will tend to move only in certain planes and thereby lose flexibility in your spine, which can cause problems when you need to twist or turn suddenly. Your body is formed in such a way that your back can bend forwards, backwards and sideways, and you should work to keep all these options open throughout your life.

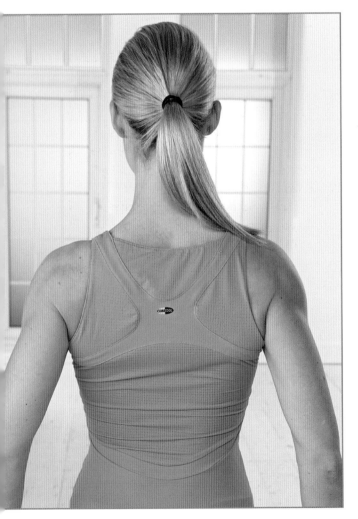

STANDING POSTURE

Whenever you are standing upright, check that your back muscles are doing what they should. Your shoulders should be back and down, not bunched up around your ears, and should contract the muscles between your shoulder blades, pulling them into your back. This will become particularly important once you start to punch and jab. Make sure your TVA is engaged (see page 32) and lift your ribcage off your waist. Take up this good, lifted posture whenever you are about to begin an exercise.

KNOW YOUR ANATOMY

The erector spinae muscles run the length of the spine and help to keep it supported, at the same time protecting the vertebrae from incorrect movements. The latissimus dorsi stabilize the torso and give shape to the upper back, while the oblique muscles of the abdominal section (see page 33) aid the spine in bending and twisting. The exercises provided here will work all these muscles, plus the rectus abdominis and TVA (see page 33).

SUPERMAN

This exercise will strengthen your erector spinae muscles. Kneel on all fours with your hands flat on the floor. Check that your back is straight, your TVA engaged (see page 32) and your weight distributed equally on knees and hands.

Slowly extend your left arm and right leg away from you, so that both are parallel with the floor. Hold for a count of 3 – you will feel your back muscles working. Release your arm and leg back down, then repeat on the other side. Repeat 10 times.

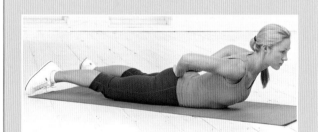

VARIATION: BACK RELIEVER

If you have back problems, start with your hands behind your back rather than by your ears.

BACK EXTENSIONS

Lie face down with your forehead touching the floor. Place your hands by your ears and keep your legs straight and together. Now lift your head and shoulders off the floor, keeping your hands in place, as high as you can manage comfortably. You will need to squeeze your buttocks as you lift. Slowly lower back down to the floor. Repeat 5 times.

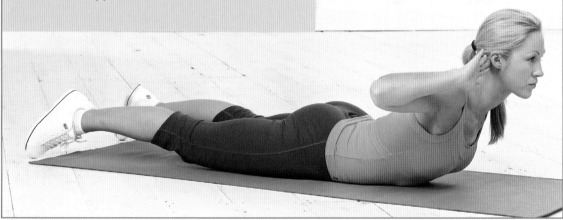

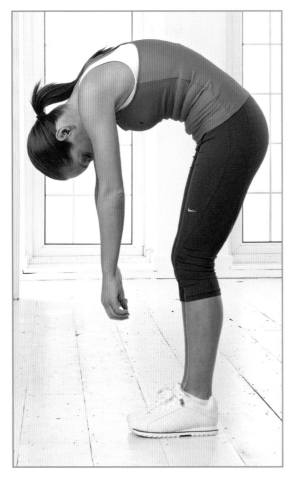

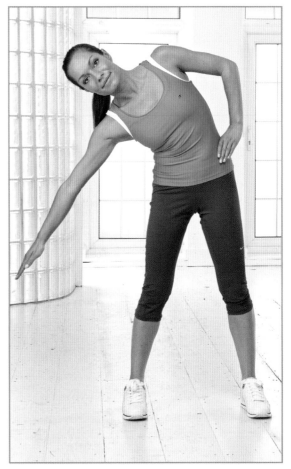

ROLL DOWN

Stand tall with your arms by your sides and feet together, legs very slightly bent. Drop your head forward on to your chest, then allow its weight to pull your upper body slowly forward so that your back is curling forward vertebra by vertebra. As you continue to curl, your arms will naturally fall forward, then your ribcage, until your hands touch the floor. At this point take a breath in and out; then, starting at your pelvis, begin to uncurl back up again vertebra by vertebra, until the last thing to straighten up is your head. Repeat 2–3 times.

SIDEWAYS LEAN

Stand with your feet just over hip width apart and your TVA engaged (see page 32). Reach your left hand up and out to the side and as you do so place your right hand on your hip. Lifting up and over (rather than collapsing), lean over to your right until your right arm is reaching to the floor. This extends the whole left side of your body. Lift back up and repeat on the other side, swapping arms as you go. Repeat 4 times on each side.

BACKWARD BEND

Your back is configured to bend backwards, and doing so will stimulate the fluid between the vertebrae and help to keep your spine supple. Stand lifted with your hands on your hips and feet hip width apart. Lift up through your ribcage and press your hips forward. As you do so, bend your upper body backwards. To start with, this move may feel quite scary, so take it steady and only bend back as far as you feel comfortable. Focus on contracting your abdominals to lift you back to upright. Repeat 4 times on each side.

stretch YOURSELF

This set of stretches allows you to work on improving your range of movement. This means that you hold each position for longer and work to stretch the muscles so that you can get progressively further. When you achieve greater flexibility you will be able to kick higher and faster, as well as move more easily in all combinations, because your body is more mobile.

SIDE SPLITS

Stretching out your inner thighs (the adductor muscles) will really improve your kicks and leg lifts.

Sit on the floor with your legs wide apart, your upper body lifted and shoulders back. Turn your knees up towards the ceiling. Lean your upper body forward and reach out – depending on your flexibility, you may be able place your hands on the floor and then work your body further forward. If you are not yet this flexible, hold on to something solid in front of you and use this to pull yourself forward. Work and hold, work and hold for a count of 15, then slowly release.

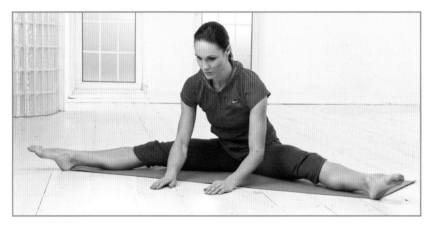

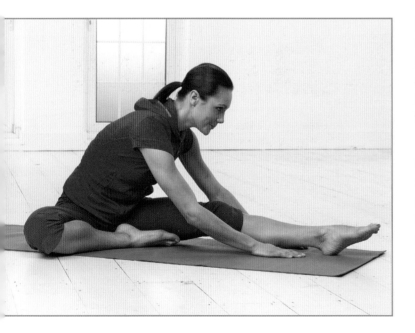

CORNER STRETCH

Stretching out your hamstrings will really increase the mobility in all your leg work. This stretch will allow you to work on lengthening your hamstring on one leg while providing a stretch in the hip and lower back on the other side.

Sit on the floor with your left leg straight out in front of you. Bend your right leg so that the knee falls out and the foot is tucked into your inner thigh. Slowly reach forward and try to press your chest towards your knee. You will feel a lengthening in the back of your thigh (hamstring muscle), and if you get over far enough you will also feel a stretch in the opposite side of your lower back. Hold for a count of 15, then repeat on the other side.

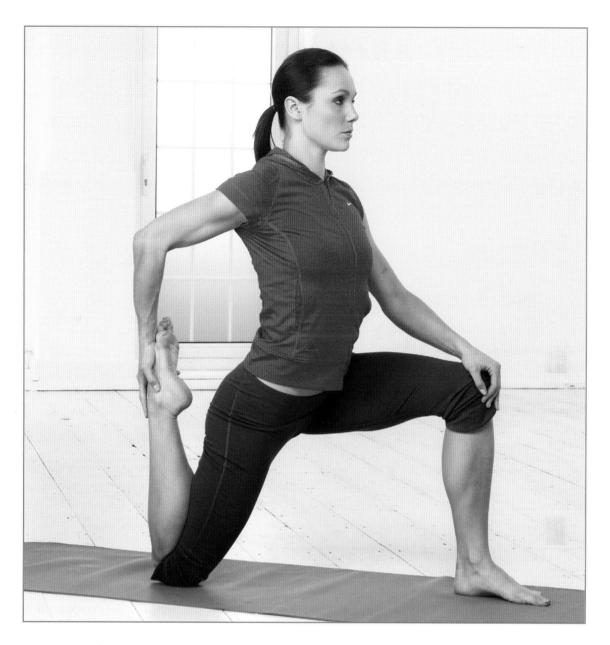

THIGH STRETCH

This exercise will help to stretch out the front of your thighs and your hip area.

Kneel on your right knee with your left foot on the floor in front, knee bent at a right angle. Lean forward on to that leg so that you can feel a stretch in your right hip. Lift up your right heel towards your buttocks, reach behind with your right hand and take hold of your foot. Pull your heel towards your buttocks for a really intense stretch! Hold for a count of 10, then release and repeat on the other side.

SAFETY FIRST
Stretch only as far as is comfortable – you should feel a stretch but no pain.

classic BOXER'S EXERCISES

There are some exercises that are traditionally associated with boxing, so now's the time to have a go at these. Work your way through the exercises described here and on the following pages, then integrate them into your conditioning routine before you start your boxing technique practice.

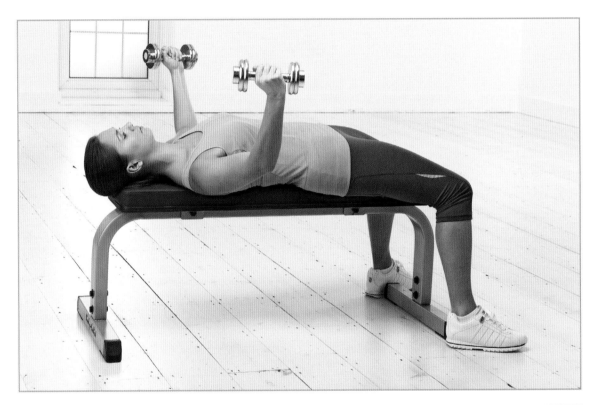

FLAT BENCH FLIES

All too often women ignore their upper body when training, yet a toned chest and arms can really enhance your shape. Boxers need a very strong upper torso and this is one of their classic exercises. You will need a pair of dumbbells – if you don't have any, use a couple of plastic bottles of water. You can also use cushions under your back and head instead of a bench.

Place the dumbbells on the floor near your bench. Lie on your back on the bench and engage your TVA (see page 32). Take a dumbbell in each hand and bend your arms at right angles. Move the arms in an arc over your body and almost touch the dumbbells together, then slowly open out to the start position. Repeat 20 times.

TECHNIQUE
✳ Keep the lower back pressed against the bench.

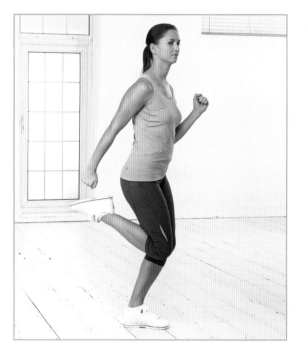

JOGGING

Whenever you can, get outside and do some jogging. Wear a pair of good jogging shoes and tracksuit trousers. Set your stopwatch, pick up your knees and jog slowly down the road. Have your head lifted and your shoulders back, and keep breathing and pumping your arms. After 5 minutes, simply turn around and jog back. Jog as slowly as you need to in order to keep going without stopping. Even if this seems really hard work at first, it pays to persist as jogging works your heart and lungs, and provides excellent fat-burning exercise. Aim to add 1 minute to your time on the way out and 1 minute on the way back, each time you jog. If you can't get outside, jog on the spot kicking up your heels behind you.

CRUNCHES

A whole set of abdominal exercises is provided on pages 32–35, but you should also know the classic boxer's crunch.

Lie on your back with your hands behind your head and your legs lifted up towards the ceiling with the ankles crossed. Now lift your head and shoulders off the floor, curving your back so that your elbows come either side of your knees.

LEVELS

Level 1 Perform 10 reps.
Level 2 Add 10 reps at every third session.
Level 3 Perform 100 reps.

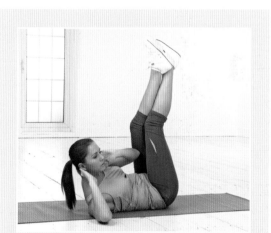

VARIATION: OBLIQUE

This variation uses the oblique muscles of your abdominal area. As you crunch up, bring your elbow towards the opposite knee so that you are twisting your body across. Then bring the other elbow across to the opposite knee before you lower.

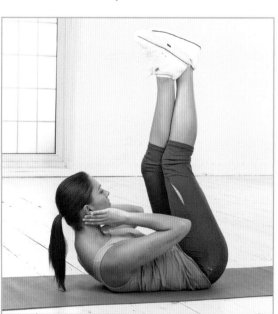

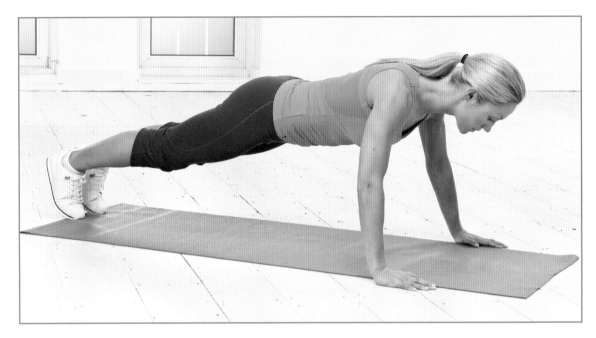

PUSH-UPS

This is another classic boxer's exercise and a great all-round toner. It will strengthen your chest, arms and abdominals.

1 To get into position, start by kneeling on all fours, then straighten your legs, lift your knees off the floor and push up into a raised position, with your hands in a wide position and toes only on the floor. Keep your head lifted, your back straight and your abdominals strong.

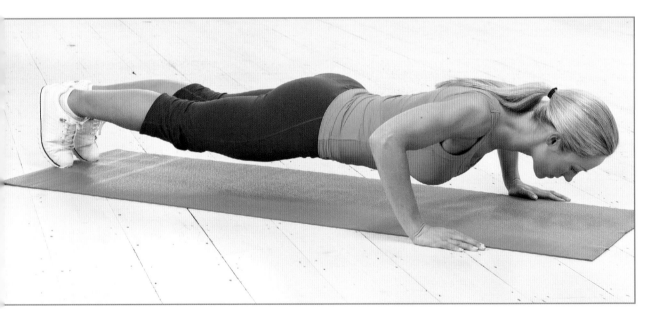

2 Now bend your arms slowly and lower your whole body so that you can touch your nose to the floor, then straighten your arms and push your body back up. Don't allow your mid-section to dip at all — try to keep your body as straight as a plank of wood. Repeat 20 times.

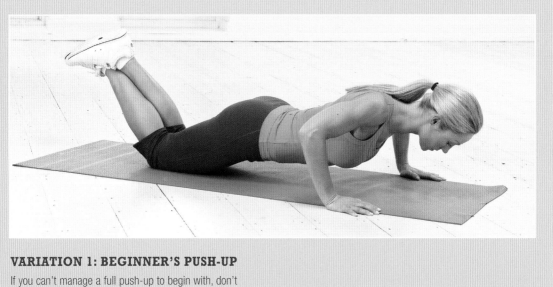

VARIATION 1: BEGINNER'S PUSH-UP

If you can't manage a full push-up to begin with, don't worry. Start on your knees (as opposed to your toes) and lower the whole body down and then up.

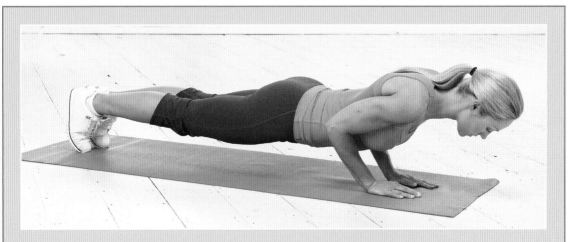

VARIATION 2: TRICEPS TONER

This version will place more emphasis on the triceps muscles (back of the upper arms), toning and shaping them nicely. Kneel on hands and knees or use the full push-up position, but place your arms in a narrower position with your elbows tucked into your ribcage. As you lower your body, bend your arms so that your elbows remain tucked in.

SKIPPING

Skipping is the boxer's staple conditioning workout, probably because it is so versatile. It can act as a warm-up or as the cardiovascular part of your regime (and become quite intense), and can also help with agility work. A skipping rope is easily flung into a bag, so if you're travelling or staying away from home you can always take one with you. You can buy a good skipping rope from any sports or fitness store. The problem for beginners is that you may keep tripping over the rope, but don't let that stop you: keep breathing, keep practising, and you will soon master the co-ordination.

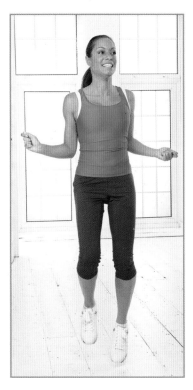

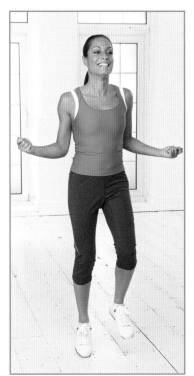

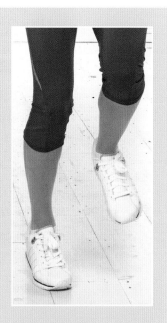

TECHNIQUE

✳ As you bounce from one foot to the other, aim to land on the ball of your foot and then roll the rest of the foot down. Keep your landing light and springy.

SHADOW SKIP

1 Stand on both feet and tuck your elbows into your sides, but bend your arms as if you are holding a skipping-rope handle in each hand. Now bounce from foot to foot as if you were jumping over the rope. Rotate your wrists as if you were flicking the rope and keep your upper torso lifted.

2 As you continue, bring your non-weightbearing foot out in front of you (not behind, as when jogging), lifting it up slightly to the ankle level of your standing foot. Aim to keep going for 2 minutes.

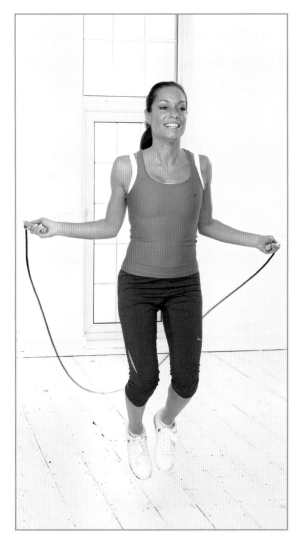

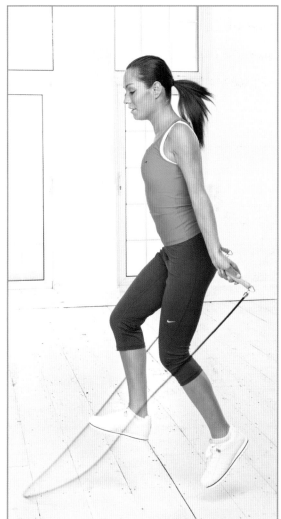

TWO-FOOTED SKIP

Now try skipping for real! Check the length of the rope: when you stand on the rope, the handles should come up to your armpits. Holding the rope, start with two-footed jumps: take off and land on both feet. Swing the rope from your wrist, keeping your elbows tucked in. Land on the balls of your feet and try to get a rhythm going. If you jump on the rope, don't worry – just untangle yourself and try again. Aim to keep going for 1 minute.

BOXER'S BOUNCE

Now aim to do the shadow skip you practised earlier, but this time with the rope. This is the real boxer's bounce! Bounce from foot to foot while swinging the rope and jumping over it. Keep the lifted foot at ankle height in front of you. Once you've got this going, you can move around your space – bouncing forwards, backwards and from side to side. When you get the rhythm of this skip you will really enjoy it. Aim to keep going for 2 minutes.

cool body, COOL MIND

After each boxing fitness session, you need to do a cool-down session. This ensures that you bring your body temperature down slowly – you'll be really warm after your warm-up, conditioning, technique and combination work!

SWORD-SWEEP ADAGE

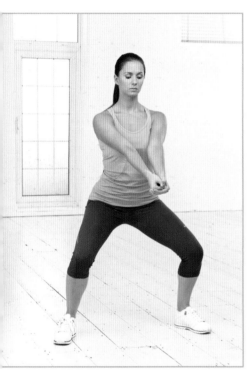
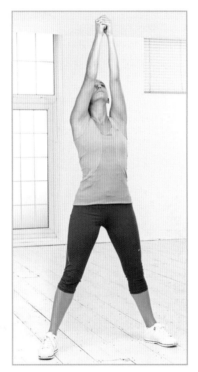
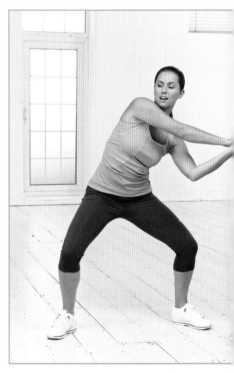

1 Use some steady, majestic music to inspire you through this section – here, adage signifies a leisurely pace. Stand with your feet 1½ hip widths apart and imagine you are holding a heavy sword in both hands. Bend your knees and drop your buttocks low to the ground as you bring the sword down slowly between your feet.

2 Lift the sword up again and bend backwards slightly as you take the sword over your head.

TECHNIQUE
* Make sure all your movements are slow and graceful.
* Keep your focus on the moment: look at the imaginary sword and move as if it were heavy and sharp.

3 Now swing the sword as if you were slicing something to your right and then to your left. Make other slow-motion sweeping and cutting movements with the sword, as you bend your body first one way and then the other. Keep the movement going for the whole piece of music.

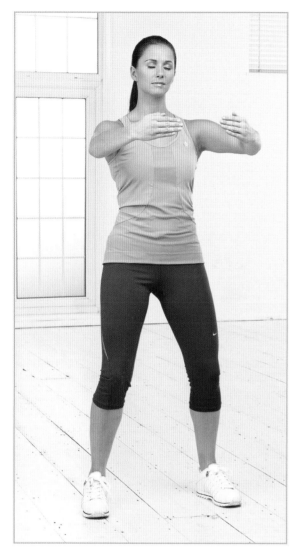

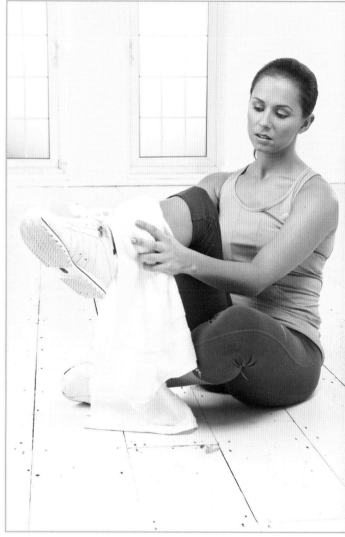

HUGGING A TREE

This is an exercise from chi kung – a Chinese practice of meditation, therapeutic movement and breathing – that will bring you to a calm place. It works with energy, and the belief that our physical and mental processes are inextricably linked together. Chi is believed to be the life force that circulates throughout the body and allowing it the smoothest route possible is the aim of many chi kung movements.

Stand with your feet 1½ hip widths apart, then round your arms and link your fingers in front of you – as if you were hugging a huge tree trunk! Inhale deeply and try to feel the roundness and thickness of the shape of the tree, even though it's not actually there. Focus your thoughts and energy on the tree and remain in this position for 10 deep breaths.

TOWEL SCRUB

Finally, before you begin your stretches, grab a towel with a good hard pile and give yourself a rub. Start at your ankles and rub the towel upwards over your calves and thighs. Use long, brisk strokes to stimulate the lymph system. Brush over your buttocks and stomach, and upwards over your arms and chest, before rubbing the back of your neck and wiping the sweat from your brow. You are now ready to stretch out your hardworked muscles.

stretch OUT

When you have worked your muscles hard, contracting and extending them, it helps to stretch them out afterwards. Stretching contributes to the cooling-down process and allows your muscles to return comfortably to their pre-exercise length.

CHEST STRETCH

This exercise focuses on stretching out your chest, shoulders and arms, which you will have used a lot in your workout.

SHOULDER STRETCH

This exercise works on your shoulders and arms, stretching the muscles just enough to be effective without strain.

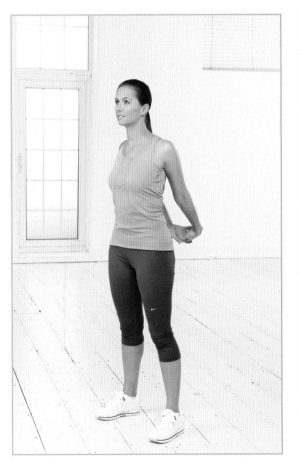

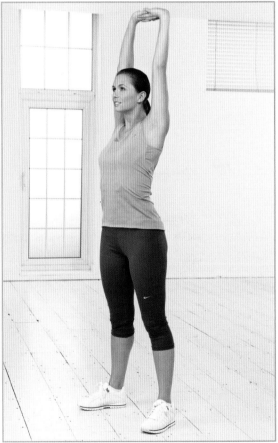

Stand with your feet hip width apart and engage your TVA (see page 32). Link your hands behind your back, pulling your shoulders back. Slowly lift up your hands behind you as far as they will go. You will feel the stretch across your chest in the pectoral muscles and also across the front of your shoulders, stretching the deltoids. Hold the stretch for a count of 10–15.

Stand with your feet hip width apart and reach both hands above your head. Link the fingers and extend the arms as you press the shoulders back behind the ears as far as you can. Hold the stretch for a count of 10–15.

When you are as far over as you think you can go, extend your left arm from behind your head out across the top of your ear. Aim for your arm to be parallel with the floor. Repeat on the other side.

SIDE STRETCH

This is a classic stretch-and-tone exercise, but here the emphasis is on the stretching out of the side of your body.

1 Stand with your feet 1½ hip widths apart and place your right hand on your hip. Lift up your left hand to the ceiling then lean to the side as far as you can. Stretch the arm to give you the impetus to lift back to upright. Work the stretch for a count of 10 by trying to get your hand progressively nearer the floor.

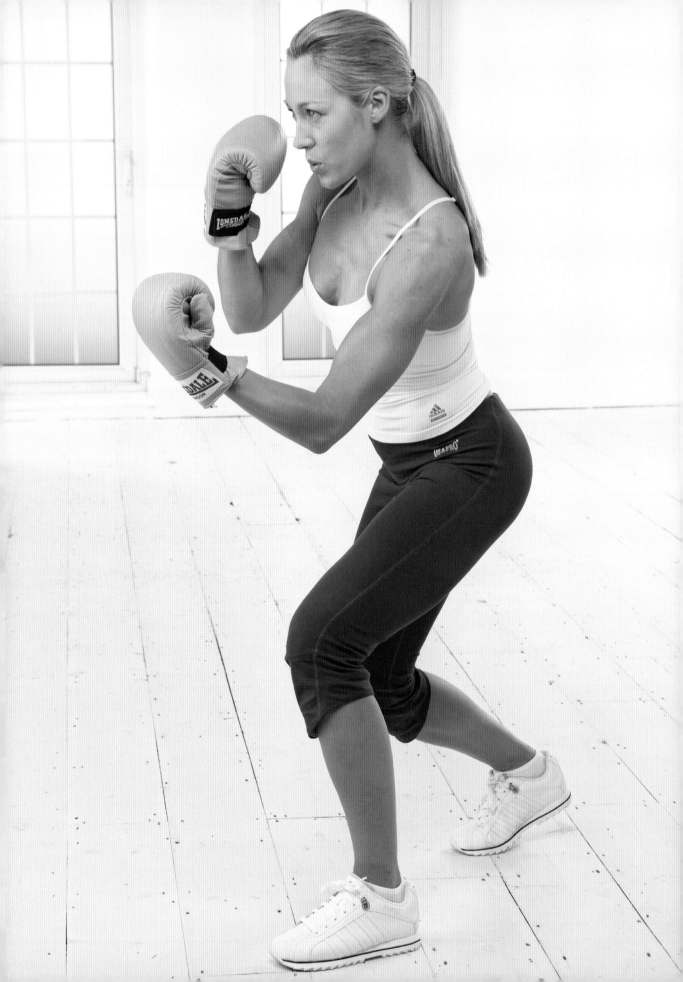

KNOCK-OUT BODY

The upper body is a much overlooked area, particularly in women. This chapter will change all that by providing you with a whole new vocabulary of punches, twists and thrusts that will shape and tone your entire upper torso. Here you will learn the basic lexicon of punches that a traditional ring boxer would use, as well as adding many other thrusts and strike moves that come from martial arts. Ducking, punching, twisting and leaning combinations will ensure that your waist and torso are challenged, leading to big improvements in your balance, flexibility and shape.

JAB

There are four main punches in boxing. The jab is the major knock-out tactic of the successful boxer: aimed correctly, with strength, it's the killer blow that will have your opponent on the floor. Think aggression and commitment: imagine the face of someone you'd dearly love to punch and go for it!

KNOCK-OUT TIPS

✳ Don't slam your punching arm straight (see page 21) – just jab and retract it.

✳ Keep your TVA engaged (see page 32) so that your arms are well supported by your torso.

✳ Expel air as you punch for increased power.

LEVELS

Level 1 Perform 5 jabs with each arm.

Level 2 Perform 10 jabs with each arm in quick succession.

Level 3 Gallop from side to side (see page 77), performing 4 jabs with your leading arm at the end of each gallop.

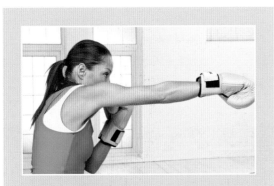

TECHNIQUE

✳ Keep your shoulder up high to protect your face. If you are really extending your arm and using your upper back for extra power, your shoulder should be up by your ear.

✳ Look down your arm as you throw the punch and return the glove to your chin fast.

✳ The power in this move comes from your legs and ribcage as you follow through.

✳ Don't swing your arm back to strike forward; the jab comes forward from your ribcage.

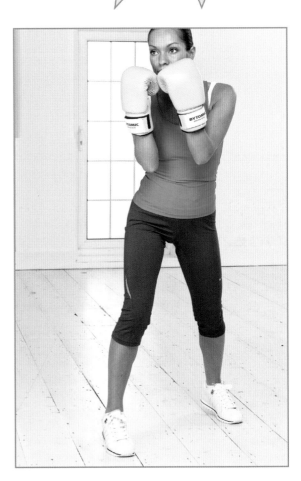

1 Start in combat stance, with your weight evenly distributed and your body sideways on to your imaginary opponent. Hold your fists up to protect your chin and your elbows tucked into your ribcage so as to protect your upper torso.

2 For a jab, you always throw the punch with your front hand. Extend your arm and rotate your fist so that the knuckles are horizontal and on top. Looking out over the first two knuckles, you punch forward, then pull your arm back into your body again.

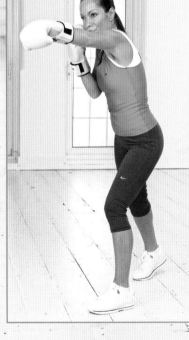

3 Perform 5 punches with one arm, then 5 with the other.

CROSS

If you were fighting a real boxing match, the only way to make the jab more effective would be to marry it with the cross punch – that way, your opponent never gets a chance! The cross is a power punch that is always thrown by the back arm and aimed at your opponent's body. All the real power comes from the back of your body as it is rotated forward.

KNOCK-OUT TIPS

* Think: weight behind the punch, move your body to power your arm.
* Focus on the body you are aiming to punch – look and aim.

LEVELS

Level 1 Perform 10 cross punches on each side, keeping them sudden and unpredictable.

Level 2 Perform a jab and a cross as fast as you can for 1 minute, maintaining your form.

Level 3 Perform 20 jab/cross combinations as you move around the room, practising both slow and fast versions.

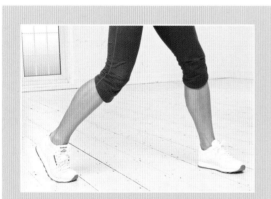

TECHNIQUE

* As you use your arm, follow through with your upper torso, twisting on the ball of your back foot.

* Your shoulder should come up to protect your chin.

* Start the movement at your foot and wind like a corkscrew to throw your weight behind the punch.

* The power in this move comes from the twist of your foot, then the turn of your waist and then your ribcage, allowing you to release your arm like a spring with no warning!

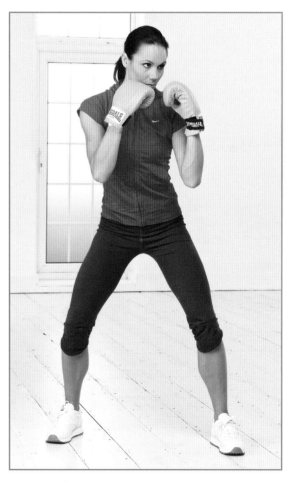

1 Position yourself in combat stance with your fists raised for protection, arms tucked into your ribcage and your TVA engaged. Start the move by twisting on the ball of your back foot.

2 Throw the punch and extend your arm across the front of your body to punch your imaginary opponent's body directly in front of you, taking care not to over-extend your arm.

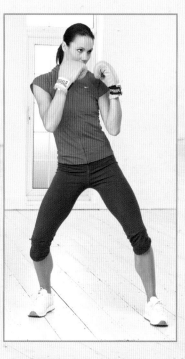

3 Spring back to stay defensive ready for the next move. Stay alert!

HOOK

This is a great move to get your assailant flailing! The punch is aimed directly at the side of the head and in a boxing match is used as the surprise element, so aim to move with killer precision and make the move snap into action.

LEVELS

Level 1 Perform 10 hooks on each side.

Level 2 Perform a jab, a cross and then a hook, 10 times on each side.

Level 3 Perform a hook to the head and then bend low to deliver a hook to the body. Repeat 10 times on each side, varying the speed from fast to lightning fast!

KNOCK-OUT TIPS

✳ Don't swing your arm back to perform the hook: keep it in close to your ribcage as you start the move.

✳ Use a vertical fist to protect your knuckles from getting hurt.

✳ Your pivoting heel always drives the punch, thereby avoiding undue pressure on your back.

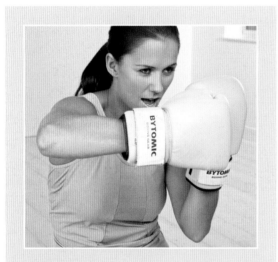

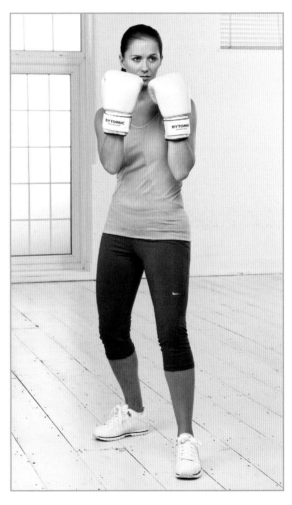

TECHNIQUE

✳ Your elbow and wrist should be at the same height and your fist vertical.

✳ The momentum comes from the twist of your upper body and feet.

✳ Punch as if you are punching through your target, not just at it.

✳ A hook can be thrown by the front or rear arm.

✳ Keep your other hand up in guard position.

1 Start in combat stance with your TVA engaged (see page 32).

2 Pivot on your back foot, twist your torso and prepare to throw a punch to the side of your imaginary opponent's head.

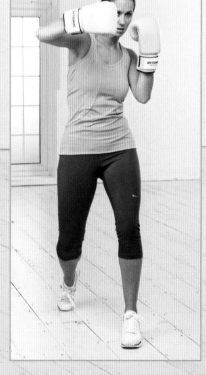

3 Twist from your back foot, keeping your punching arm bent at a right angle and elbow lifted as you swing your arm around the side of your opponent, to hit the side of the head.

UPPERCUT

In boxing, the uppercut can be lethal. To deliver this punch correctly, you need to be up close to your imaginary opponent so as not to leave yourself off balance. You will need to dip low and bring a driving force upwards.

LEVELS

Level 1 Perform 10 uppercuts with each arm.

Level 2 Perform a jab, a cross and then an uppercut, 10 times on each side.

Level 3 Perform really low uppercuts so that you have to squat down, then come up higher to aim for your imaginary opponent's chin. Alternate levels for 10 times on each side.

KNOCK-OUT TIPS

✸ Think power: coil your body like a spring and hit out fast, furious and upwards.

✸ Remember to keep spiralling your legs and turning your ribcage. This will keep your spine safe, prevent you over-stressing your arms *and* give you a great torso workout!

1 For this move you can be in combat stance (as shown) or forward stance. Bounce lightly on your feet a little and keep your fist up close to your chin.

2 Now bend your knees and bend down further in the lunge so as to give you more leverage.

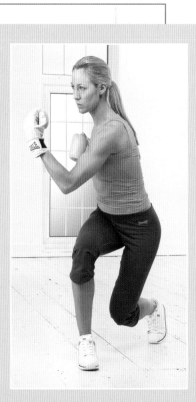

VARIATION: TWISTED PUNCH

To perform the uppercut from a side angle simply rotate your body, spiralling your legs inwards to create momentum, and then punch upwards.

3 Bring your arm up vertically as you punch upwards – as if trying to hit someone under the chin – moving your body, not just your arm. Bend low and drive the movement from your rear hip. Rotate your body to create momentum as you punch.

SPEEDBALL

The speedball is a lightweight ball on a strong spring that is used in boxing training to build reaction time and mobility in the arms. With shadow speedball – that is, without the equipment – you are working on moving your arms quickly and building stamina and co-ordination for your upper torso.

LEVELS

Level 1 Keep speedballing fast for 1 minute.

Level 2 Increase the speed and aggression, again for 1 minute – knock it out!

Level 3 Move around as you speedball with your upper half and dance with your lower half, for 1 minute.

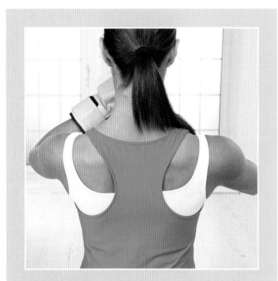

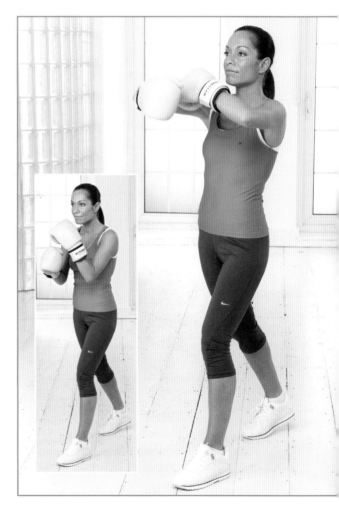

TECHNIQUE

✳ Keep your shoulder blades retracted as you revolve your arms.

✳ Keep your TVA engaged throughout (see page 32) as a strong base to support the movement in your upper torso.

1 Stand in combat stance with your fists raised in front of your face. Pretend you are hitting a ball knuckle over knuckle, very fast. Revolve one fist over the other as you hit the ball.

3 Now move the ball to the side of you, so that you are hitting to one side. Lean forward and then back as you continue to move your arms.

2 Now revolve your fists towards you as you hit the ball.

torso TRIALS

You have now learned the major punches from the traditional sport of boxing. Shortly, you will also learn some martial-arts based moves you can do with the upper body. First, however, you need to consolidate your torso work. As you now know, a punch involves not just your arm but your whole body. Impetus comes from your foot, leg and the spiralling of your body to produce energy and action. The torso is a key mover in boxing fitness and the torso-twisting moves shown here will really loosen up your mid-section.

DUCK AND DIVE

This is a classic boxing manoeuvre that is used defensively to avoid punches.

RIBCAGE JIVE

This is a practice exercise to get your torso moving and increase your self-protection mode. It will give you great flexibility in your mid-section and really tone your waist.

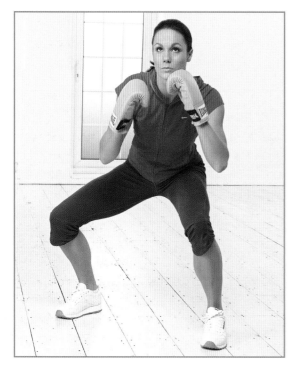

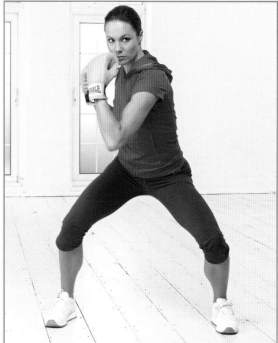

Stand with your feet 1½ hip widths apart. Throw some of the punches you have just mastered: a jab, a hook and an uppercut. Now imagine your opponent is about to hit you back – and duck! Bend your knees, squat low and circle your upper torso underneath the impending blow. Practise dodging blows from both the left and right sides.

1 Start in forward stance with your fists up to protect your chin, elbows tucked into your ribcage and knees slightly bent. As you gradually squat lower, twist your upper torso and bring your left elbow forward.

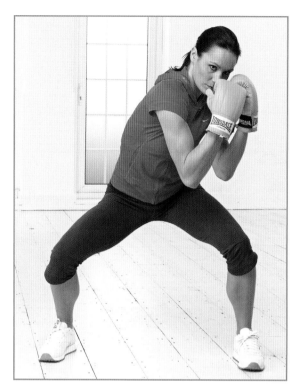

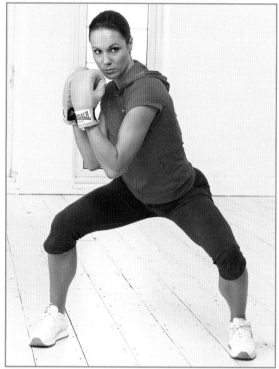

2 Now twist the other way to bring your right elbow forward, moving from your ribcage.

3 Practise sinking low and rising higher as you twist your upper body first to one side and then the other.

TWIST IT FURTHER

To really work your twists, perform this stretch from time to time to help develop your mobility.

Sit on the floor with your right foot crossed over your straight left leg. Press your foot into the floor as you turn your torso in towards your knee. If you can, place your left elbow behind your right knee; if not, hold on to your knee with your left hand. Use this position to work the twist so that you can turn further around to the back. Remain in position for a count of 5, the whole time working to twist further. You will feel the twist/stretch in your ribcage, waist and spine areas. Release and repeat on the other side.

martial arts MAGIC

Now that you've got the boxing moves under your belt (as it were!), you can add in some variety with a little martial arts magic. Check out these moves to add to your repertoire.

KNOCK-OUT TIPS

✳ Think: forward, devastating contact – thrust those fists!

✳ As with all arm moves, don't over-extend your arm joints.

LEVELS

Level 1 Perform 5 stacked punches.

Level 2 Increase the speed and aggression, and perform 5 stacked punches.

Level 3 Bounce down and jab, straighten and cross, then straighten and stack punch, 3 times.

STACKED PUNCH

This is a fun move that feels as if you are delivering a killer blow to your imaginary opponent. Use your abdominal strength to provide a firm base from which to thrust your arms forward with aggression!

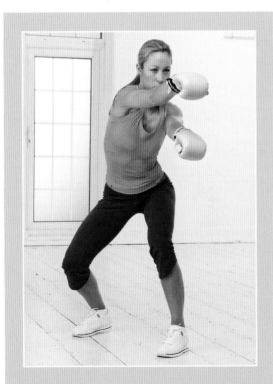

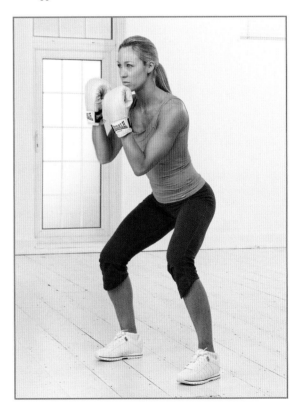

TECHNIQUE

✳ Bounce into the move. Start with straight legs then bend into the squat, stack punch and straighten, throwing the arms out towards your opponent.

1 Start in a bounce stance with your feet 1½ hip widths apart, TVA engaged (see page 32) and upper body lifted with shoulder blades retracted. Have your arms tucked in by your ribcage and fists ready at your chin. Your knees will bend and straighten as you deliver the move.

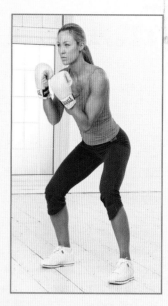

3 Draw your arms back in again and resume the bounce moving slightly from side to side.

2 Bend your legs, then thrust your arms out in front of you, aiming for your imaginary opponent's sternum with your fists stacked one above the other.

KNOCK-OUT TIPS

✳ This move is pure aggression – *stab* that elbow to knock your imaginary opponent sideways!

✳ Even though this move is aggressive, keep it light and allow your elbow to rebound after it meets its target.

ELBOW KICK

This is your chance to really give someone you don't like the elbow!

LEVELS

Level 1 Perform 10 elbow kicks on each side.

Level 2 Perform the sideways variation 5 times on each side.

Level 3 Climb the ladder: elbow right and left, starting low down and gradually getting higher and higher, 5 times on each side.

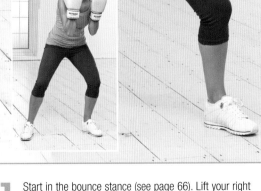

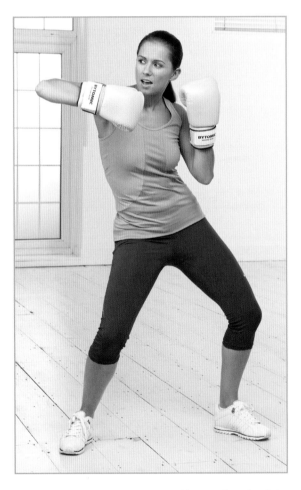

1 Start in the bounce stance (see page 66). Lift your right elbow up to horizontal.

2 Keeping your abdominals strong, jab your elbow sharply to your right – as if you were knocking someone in the eye!

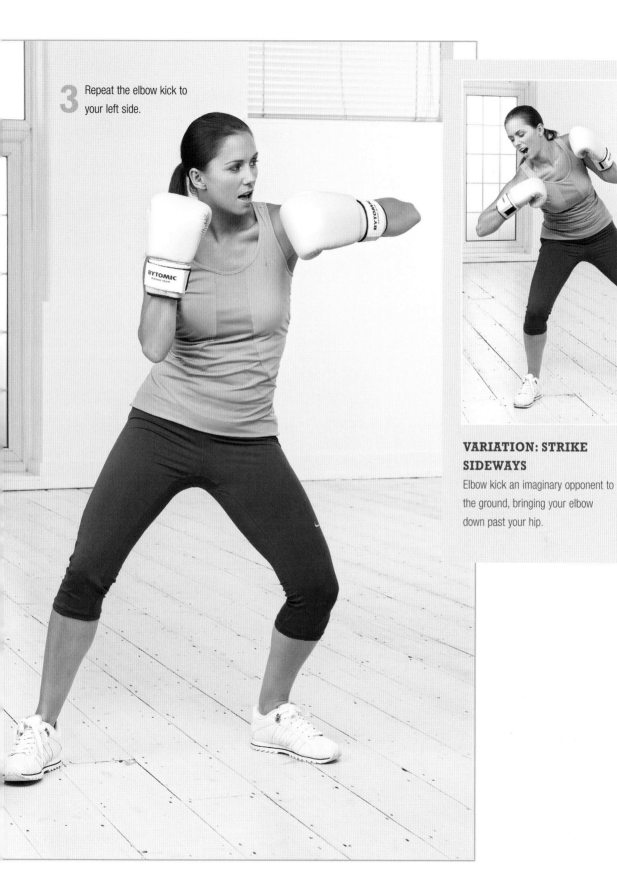

3 Repeat the elbow kick to your left side.

VARIATION: STRIKE SIDEWAYS

Elbow kick an imaginary opponent to the ground, bringing your elbow down past your hip.

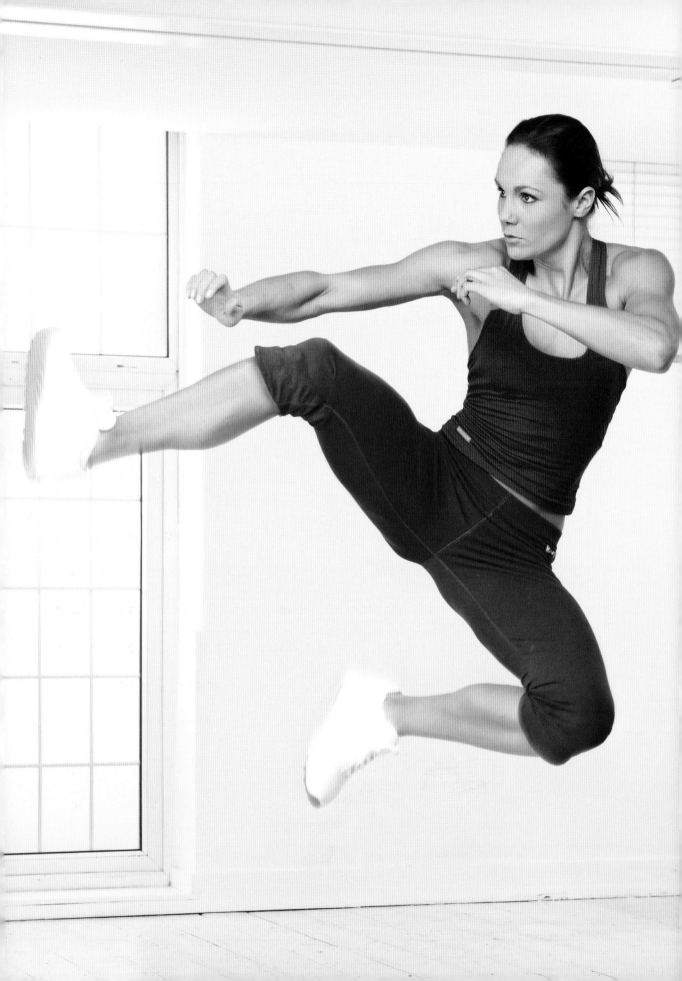

KICK-PERFECT LEGS

Balance and agility are two of the key areas covered in this chapter. Balance is very important for a boxer, who always has to be upright and ready to move in any direction. It's also important for performing the range of kicks you are going to learn later, so that you can deliver that devastating contact exactly where you want it. Agility is your ability to move quickly, safely and nimbly around a space so that you can change direction, skip, jump or run whenever you need to. Add all these aspects together and you will become a fighting force to be reckoned with!

balancing ACT

Before you attempt the legwork in this chapter, there is some additional conditioning to be done. The first of the two important elements of lower body work is balance, and the following exercises will help you master the art of balance so that you feel secure and powerful on one leg as well as two.

YOGA HOLD

This balance move is derived from the ancient art of yoga. When you first practise it you may find that you constantly fall out of balance and can't stay on one leg for any length of time. That's fine – just keep at it. Don't allow yourself to grab your toes until you can maintain the balance. Wriggle around to stay in balance, and as you keep practising you will suddenly notice that you can stay on one leg for much longer.

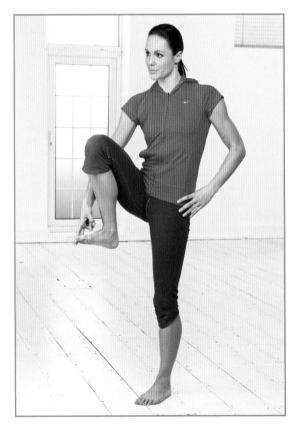

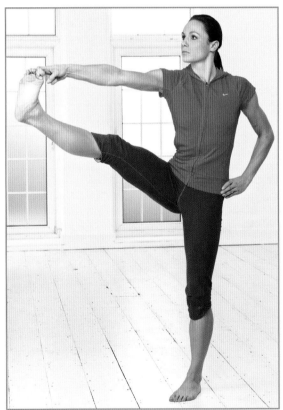

1 Stand with your feet together, body lifted and TVA engaged (see page 32). Now slowly lift your right foot off the ground and try to stay balanced.

2 Lift up your foot so that you can hook the fingers of your right hand around your big toe. Straighten up your body and leg as much as you can and hold for a count of 10. Return to the start position and repeat the move with your other leg.

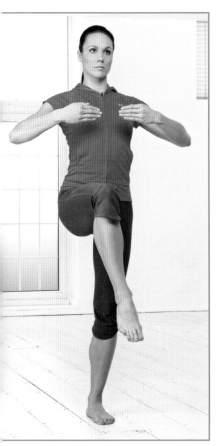

BOXER'S ADAGE

Once you start to master the basics of balance, you can develop your practice to rehearse some of the kick moves you will be learning shortly.

1 Stand with your feet together, body lifted and TVA engaged (see page 32). Now slowly lift your right foot until it is by your left knee. Bend your arms, lift your elbows and place your hands in front of your chest.

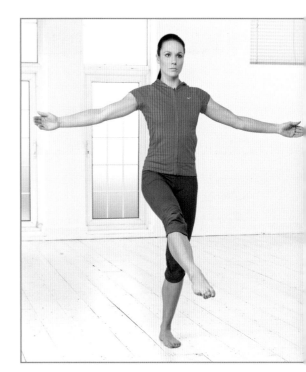

2 Slowly extend your right leg in front of you and, if you can, lean back slightly as you extend your arms out to each side for balance.

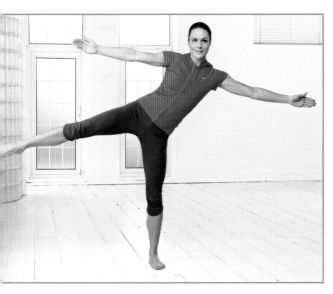

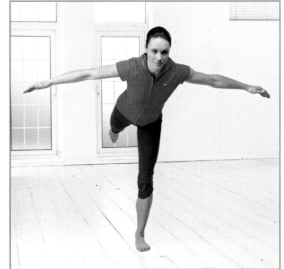

3 Now bring your arms and leg back to the starting position – you're still standing on one leg – and then extend the same leg out to the side. Lean to the opposite side as you lengthen your leg and extend your arms out to each side again.

4 Bring your arms and leg back to the starting position and then extend the same leg out behind you. Lean your body forward and extend your arms out to each side. Bring your arms and leg back to the starting position. Repeat the whole sequence with your left leg.

THROW AND CATCH

This move is designed specifically to help with your roundhouse kick (see pages 84–85). It will also improve your flexibility so practise it regularly. Make sure you have already warmed up before you perform this move, using some of the conditioning exercises on pages 28–31 and some of the stretches on pages 40–41.

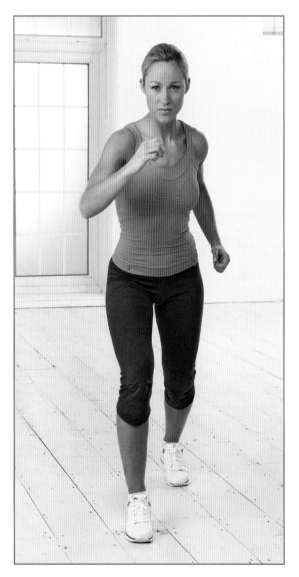

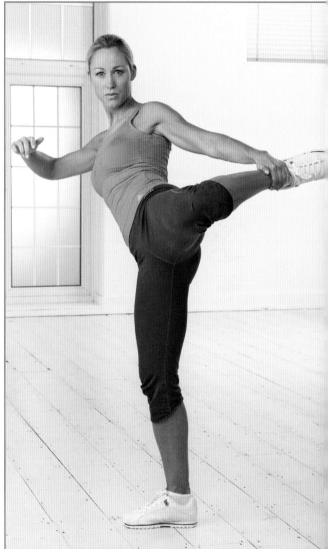

1 Stand with your feet together, body lifted and TVA engaged (see page 32). Take a step forward with your right leg and as you do so lift your left leg so that the hip-to-thigh line is straight and your calf is curled back behind you.

2 Catch your left shin with your left hand and hold for a moment with your knee and foot horizontal, then release back down. Stay balanced if you can – don't allow the leg to pull you off balance. Make the move fast and percussive (eventually you will turn this into a roundhouse kick). Now perform the sequence with your right leg, and repeat once more on each side.

SUMO SQUAT

This move works on both your flexibility and your balance. You will feel the stretch on your adductor muscles (inner thighs) as you lift your leg and this will test your balancing skills as your throw your weight to each side.

2 Now bounce lower, swing your weight to one side as you tip over and lift the other leg. Hold for a moment, keeping your abdominals working to hold your position and keep breathing. Release your leg down and swing your weight to perform the move on the other side. Repeat once more on each side.

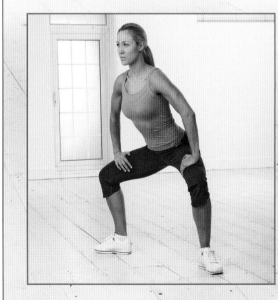

1 Take up a wide, deep squat position with your hands resting on your thighs and lower your buttocks to the level of your knees to feel the stretch across your inner thighs.

moving IT

Part of the discipline of boxing fitness is to keep moving – in other words, agility. The more you keep moving, the more you will exercise your heart and lungs and increase your cardiovascular fitness. This will improve your energy levels and reduce body fat. Boxers need to keep moving as much as they can: just remember Muhammad Ali's refrain, 'I float like a butterfly, sting like a bee!'.

ALI SHUFFLE

Whenever you are practising your punches, try to get into the habit of staying on your toes and keeping moving.

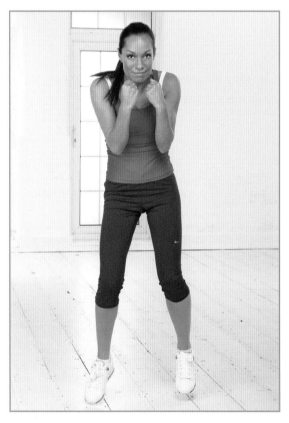

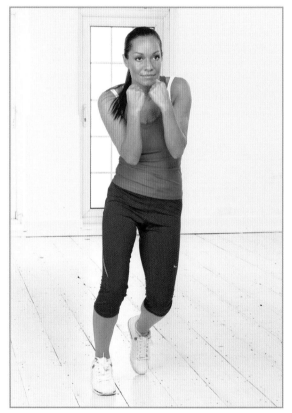

1 Keeping your hands in guard position and your TVA engaged (see pages 20 and 32), bounce from foot to foot on your toes and on your heels.

2 Once you have got a feel for this, try bouncing to one side of your space, then change direction and bounce to the next side, and so on all the way around. Try Ali shuffling backwards and forwards, then to one side and then the other. You can also combine this move with the duck and dive moves on page 64.

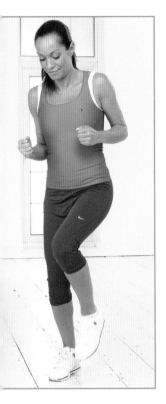

JOG AND SKIP

While not something you'd see in the boxing ring, boxers always practise jogging and skipping for stamina (see pages 43 and 46–47). During your boxing practice, whenever you can, jog on the spot for a minute or so in between moves or move into a shadow skip (no rope). This will lift your heart rate and tone your leg muscles.

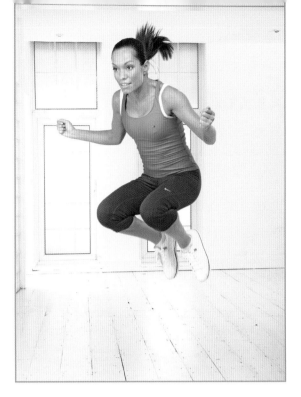

1 You can also try running really fast on the spot for 30 seconds.

2 Imagine you are doing double rope skips – you need to jump high enough to allow the rope to pass under your feet twice before you land.

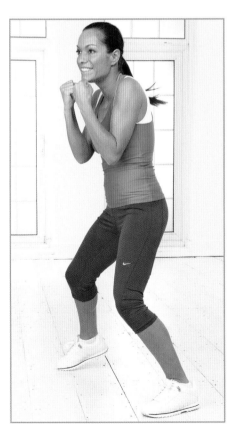

GALLOP

This is not a move used in boxing but it will get you around the space, which is what you need to keep your heart and lungs working as hard as your muscles.

In between punches or punch combinations, try galloping sideways from one side of your space to the other, keeping your knees well bent and aiming to stay low to the ground. Keep your fists up in guard position.

READY TO KICK!

You are now ready to move on to learn some of the fundamental martial arts kicks. These are great fun and will have you looking like a Kung Fu expert in no time! Practise slowly at first and then build up to speed as you become more familiar with the moves.

While you are learning, keep in mind that not all the kicks use the same method: for example, the front, side and back kicks utilize a full leg extension, while in the roundhouse kick just the lower leg is extended for that quick killer blow, then folded in and lowered.

Before attempting any kicks, you must make sure you stretch out your legs first. Performing percussive moves like these that stretch the back and sides of the legs could cause injury unless you warm up properly first (see pages 28–31).

front KICK

The front kick is just what it says. Aim your power out in front of you – you can aim high or low, but the power comes from the leg and is delivered through the heel.

LEVELS

Level 1 Perform the front kick slowly, keeping your balance throughout, 5 times on each side.

Level 2 Perform the kick faster, and use the variation if possible, 5 times on each side.

Level 3 Move the kick around your space using the Ali shuffle, completing 3–4 circuits.

KNOCK-OUT TIP

Really see your opponent in front of you. Aim your knee at where you want your kick to make contact. Wherever you aim your knee is where your foot will land.

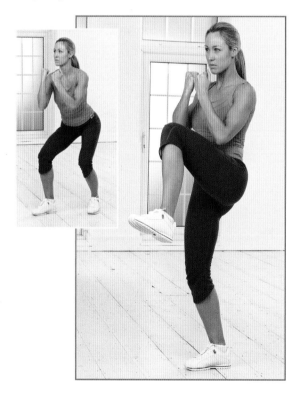

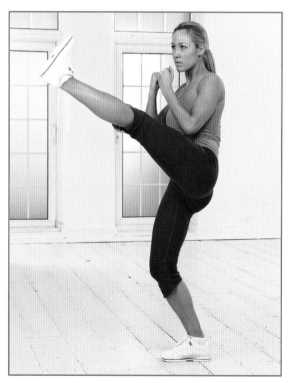

1 Start in the combat stance, fighting foot behind. Even though here you will be fighting with your legs, you still need to keep your fists up to protect your face. There are four parts to a kick and you always work through these. First is the chamber: push off your back foot and lift up your back (fighting) knee so that your thigh is in front of your stomach. Stay balanced on your supporting leg.

2 Next comes the extension: extend your leg sharply and kick – make imaginary contact – with the heel. You should push your leg straight out from the hip through the thigh to the heel. As you improve, you can try to kick the same spot each time.

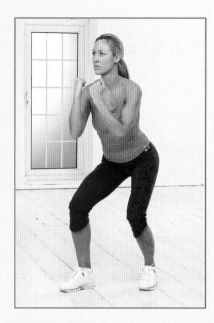

4 Finally, the placement: place your foot back down on the floor in combat stance once again.

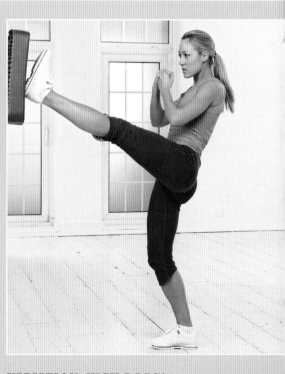

VARIATION: KICK A BAG!

If you have the opportunity to use a boxing bag or focus pad, front kick the bag.

3 Now the recoil: once you have made contact, quickly bend your leg back into the chamber position.

side KICK

This is another essential kick to add to your armoury. It enables you to devastate any attacker who comes at you from right or left by kicking out to the side. Try out the different versions provided here and on pages 82–83 – one uses the front leg for the kick and the other the back – to become a real expert.

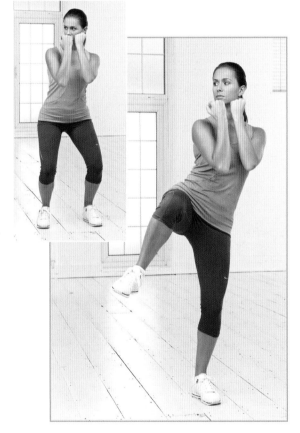

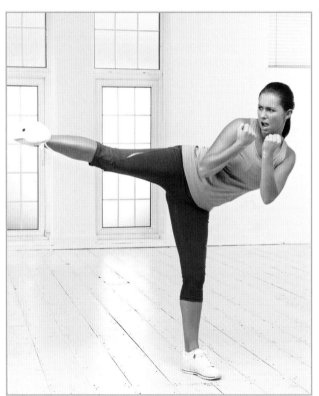

1 You can start in either forward or combat stance. Chamber: lift your front knee, keeping it close to your body and remaining balanced on your supporting leg. At this point the kick could look like a front kick or a side kick. In order to throw the side kick, first tilt your hip to lift your buttock.

2 Extension: push your whole leg out from the hip. The leg should feel as if it is extending sideways with the heel very slightly behind you. You can practise side kicking high up on your imaginary opponent's body, aiming for the head, and lower down, aiming for the knee. Try always to have your heel – with which you make contact – higher than your toes, and your knee facing forward so that you are able to push your leg straight.

3 Recoil: once you have made contact, quickly bend your leg back into the chamber position and re-centre your hips.

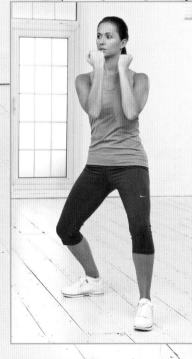

4 Placement: place your foot back down in combat stance, ready to repeat the sequence with your other leg. Repeat 5 times on each side.

spinning SIDE KICK

This is a similar technique to the side kick (see pages 80–81), but this time the kick comes from your back leg. In this move you are performing a half turn of your whole body each time.

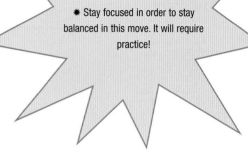

KNOCK-OUT TIP

✴ Stay focused in order to stay balanced in this move. It will require practice!

LEVELS

Level 1 Repeat 5 times on each side.

Level 2 Perform a side kick followed by a spinning side kick, 5 times.

Level 3 Gallop into a side kick, then perform a spinning side kick. Repeat on the other side.

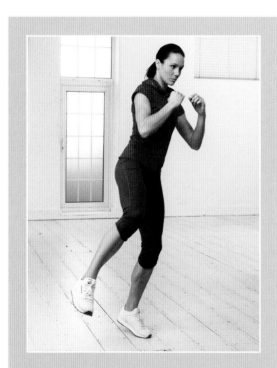

TECHNIQUE

✴ Pivot on your toe when you perform a turning kick to help you avoid any risk of injury.

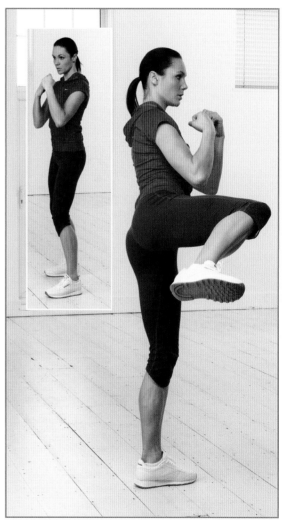

1 Start in combat stance with your left leg forward. Chamber: pivot on your left toe, push off your right leg and swing your right knee up and around to the right.

2 Extension: extend your right leg sharply to kick, making contact with your heel.

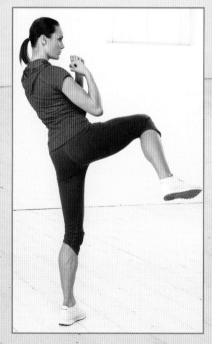

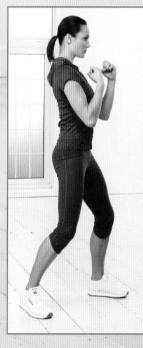

3 Recoil: once you have made contact, quickly bend your leg back into the chamber position, turning back around.

4 Placement: place your right foot back down in its original position behind. Repeat the whole sequence using your left leg to kick.

roundhouse KICK

This is a 'round the side' type of kick that is great for catching your opponent unawares! It also uses a different chamber and extension position to the kicks you have learned already, so follow the instructions carefully.

KNOCK-OUT TIPS

✻ You are kicking and making contact with the top of the foot, so keep the energy extending right through to your toes.

✻ If you're feeling the tightness in your hips, take the kick lower until you have improved your flexibility.

✻ Remember to keep breathing.

LEVELS

Level 1 Perform a roundhouse kick 5 times on each side.

Level 2 Perform a roundhouse kick followed by a side kick, 5 times.

Level 3 Kick low then high, left leg then right leg, 10 times.

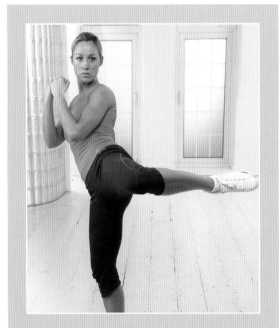

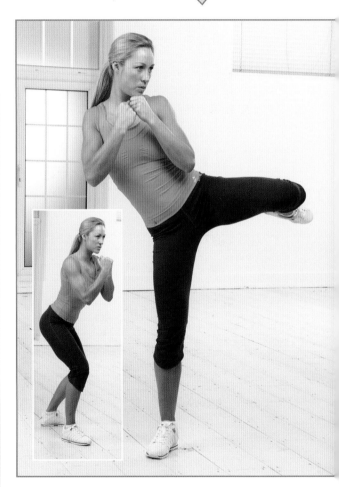

TECHNIQUE

✻ Make sure you know the difference between the knee-up chamber position for the front and side kicks (see pages 78–83) and the extended hip position for the roundhouse kick. The power in this kick comes from flicking the leg, not pushing it out.

1 Start in combat stance with your right leg forward. Chamber: gallop your back foot in and lift your left leg. This time the leg is lifted so that the hip-to-thigh line is straight and the calf is curled back behind you (see page 74).

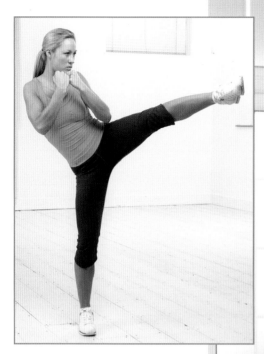

2 Extension: extend your lower leg to make contact with the top of the foot, pointing your toes.

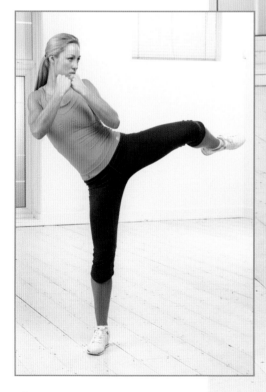

3 Recoil: curl your left leg back behind you.

4 Placement: place your left foot back down in the combat stance. Repeat the whole sequence using your right leg to kick.

back KICK

This is another leg extension kick that allows you to stab your opponent with your heel. Kicking backwards may seem counter-intuitive, but it allows you to protect your face and deliver an unexpected kick at the same time. Leaning forward as you deliver the kick allows you to stay balanced and extend your leg sharply, while spinning around to the front afterwards protects you from unexpected attack.

LEVELS

Level 1 Perform a back kick 10 times on each side.
Level 2 Perfect your aim: perform a back kick low down, then another up high, then a third at mid-level.
Level 3 Try combining all the kicks you've learned so far.

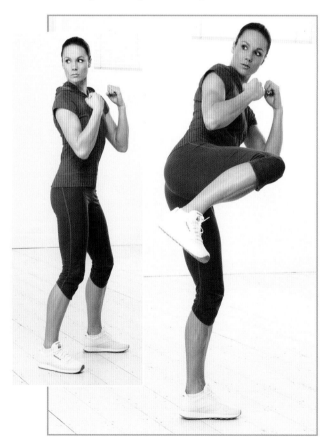

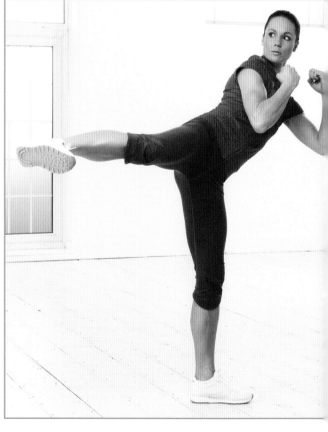

1 Start in combat stance with your left leg forward. Look behind you! Chamber: hop into the chamber position, pulling up your right leg so that your knee is close to your chest.

2 Extension: Lean forward and extend your right leg behind you to kick with the heel.

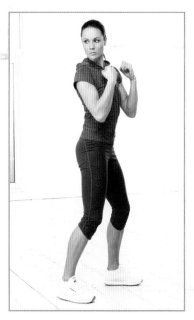

4 Placement: place your right foot back down in combat stance.

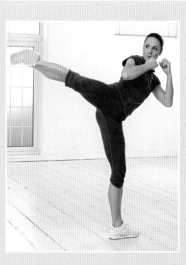

3 Recoil: bring your right leg back into the chamber position.

VARIATION: HIGH KICK

Start with a lower kick and work towards a higher kick as you increase your balance and suppleness. Start by aiming at your opponent's knee and then work up to the waist and finally the shoulder.

jump KICK

You have now learned almost all the punches and kicks you need to put together a really feisty routine. But just before you get going, here is another kick-ass move to try!

LEVELS

Level 1 Speed up the move: lift your knee (from behind) and immediately jump kick your leg forward.
Level 2 Perform the move as one smooth whole.
Level 3 Try the whole move on the other leg.

KNOCK-OUT TIPS

✹ This move takes skill: you'll need to be aware of controlling your balance for the first knee lift.

✹ Think 'explosion!' as you snap your leg into the front kick.

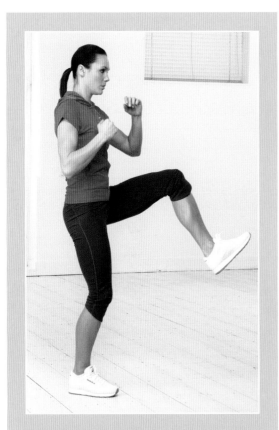

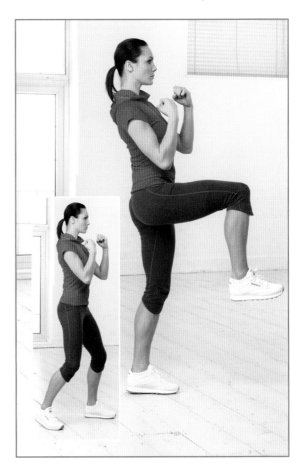

TECHNIQUE
✹ The kick itself is a front kick, so don't forget the chamber and then the extension.

1 Start in combat stance with your left foot forward. Chamber: lift your back (right) leg into a knee lift *in front* and hold.

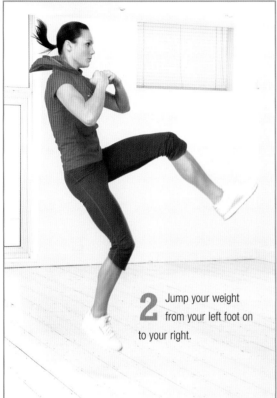

2 Jump your weight from your left foot on to your right.

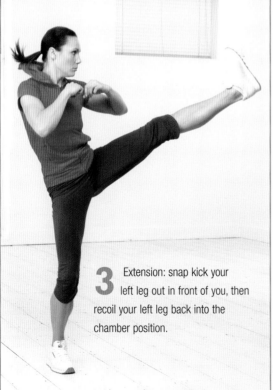

3 Extension: snap kick your left leg out in front of you, then recoil your left leg back into the chamber position.

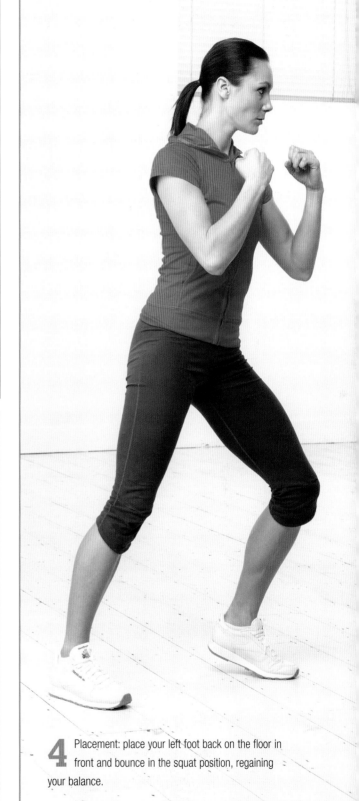

4 Placement: place your left foot back on the floor in front and bounce in the squat position, regaining your balance.

jumping BACK KICK

This is an advanced move you can have a go at for fun.
It's a kick that happens in mid-air while you jump.

LEVELS

Level 1 Perform the jump only, 5 times.
Level 2 Perform the whole move, turning one way and then the other.
Level 3 Perform a jab, a cross, a side kick and then a jumping back kick.

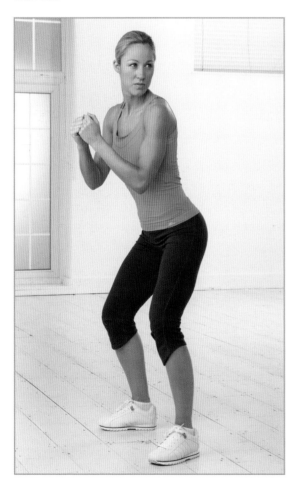

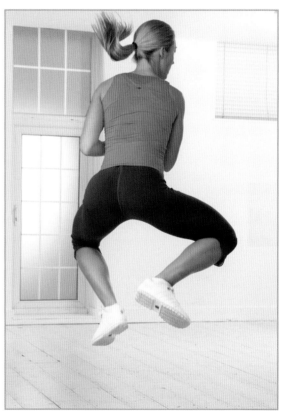

1 Start in combat stance with your left foot forward, but with your legs hip width apart in a low squat. First, practise the jump. Take off and whip your head and shoulders around in a half-turn. Your whole body should turn, your legs should be tucked up and you should land with your knees bent, facing in the opposite direction. Chamber: now jump in a half-turn again but land with one leg further behind, in a lunge position.

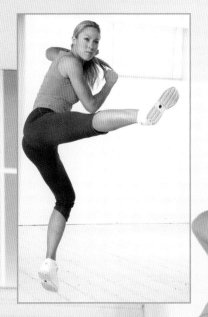

2 Extension: you now need to add the kick before you land. Jump up and half turn, and as you do so shoot out one leg fast in a back kick behind you.

3 Recoil: quickly bend your leg back in before you land.

4 Placement: you should land on one leg, quickly followed by the other – make sure you bend your knees to absorb the impact.

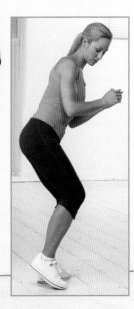

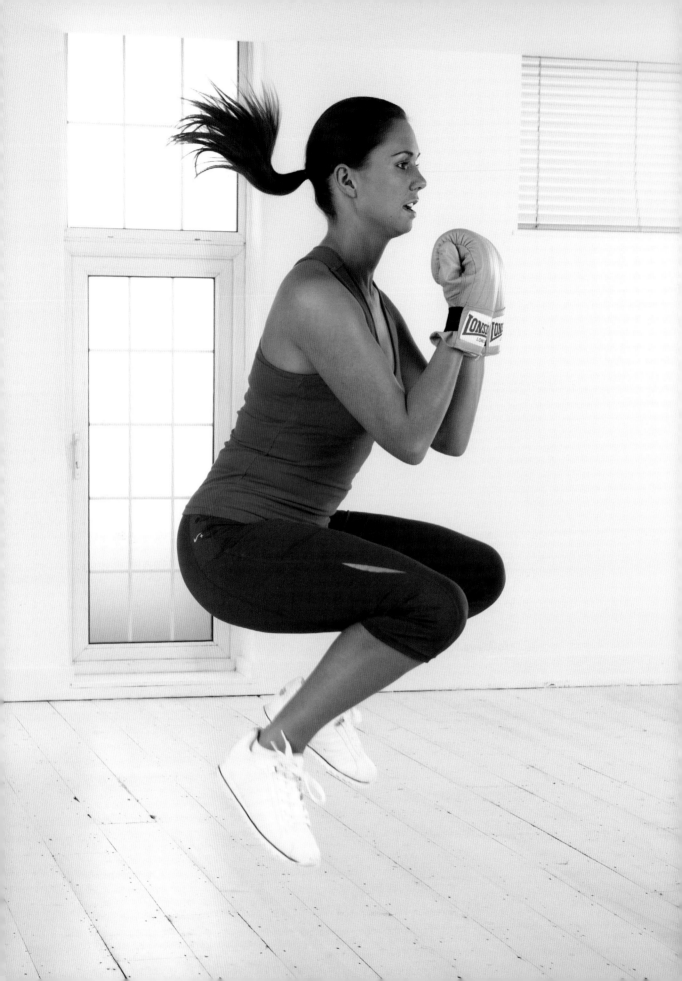

FIGHT FIT

You now have plenty of ammunition for a fantastic workout and are ready to try some combinations. The workouts you'll find on the following pages are merely suggestions for putting together the moves you have learned. There is no right or wrong way to team up all the punches, kicks and footwork you know: if you were in a boxing match or kick-boxing bout you would put them together in whatever way would keep you unscathed and hurt your opponent most. Try out some of the suggestions that follow and see how they feel, but make up your own too. Put on some inspiring music, bounce around and start throwing kicks and punches!

routine MATTERS

When it comes to trying new things, each of us has our own approach. Some like to read the manual from start to finish before they begin, others prefer to dip in and out and work through short sections at intervals. This plan is a good starting point for establishing your own routine.

12-WEEK STARTER PLAN

With boxing fitness, it's essential that you read the safety instructions given throughout this book and learn how to practise the various moves without strain. After that, it's fine to pick and choose exercises from different sections of the book – ideally, you should work out for at least 30 minutes, three times a week. However, if you want a balanced starter programme that will produce outstanding results in 12 weeks, you will find a structured week-by-week plan laid out for you on pages 96–101.

The plan is designed to guide you in building up a full and varied boxing fitness routine as you progress and learn new moves. Week by week, moves are added for you to master and extend your conditioning work and technique, so that by week 12 you will be proficient in all the key punches and kicks, as well as the other moves that make up a routine.

BEATING BOREDOM

One of the greatest barriers to successful exercising is boredom, and boxing fitness is no exception. It is very difficult to maintain your initial enthusiasm for an exercise regime once it becomes routine. To counteract this problem and keep you motivated while ensuring you make steady, sustained progress, a number of different approaches and routines are provided throughout this chapter. They range from quick wonder workouts that can be completed in just a few minutes, to challenging circuits and exercise pyramids that will really get your body moving and working hard. There is something for everyone, so whatever your level of skill and fitness you can make a start on getting boxing fit – right now!

REMEMBER

* Always warm up thoroughly before starting your workout so that you are at your best.
* Whenever you exercise, keep in mind all the safety points you have learned.
* Add variety by sometimes practising with a friend holding focus pads.
* Always cool down when you have finished.

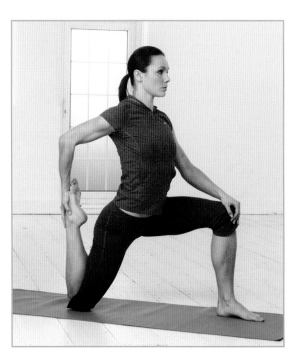

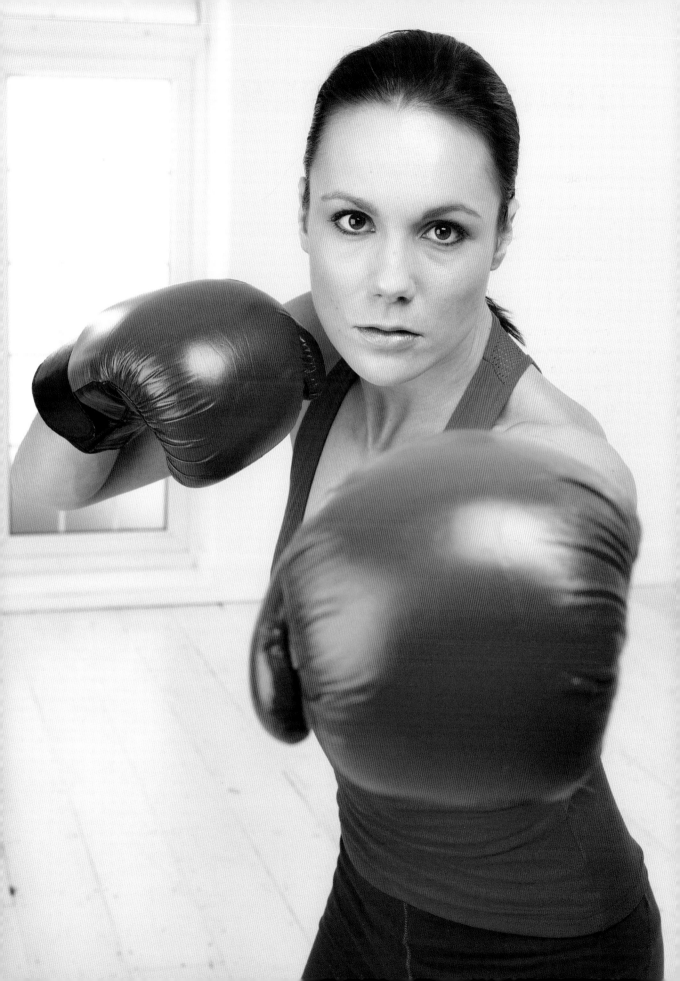

12-week STARTER PLAN

Use the combinations to put some movement between your practice kicks and punches: the travelling moves allow you to change direction and work your way around or across your space. Speedball (from week 5) will help you to bend left and right, forwards and back. Aim to exercise on 3 days per week, with at least 1 rest day between sessions. Your technique practice should take about 20 minutes, the full session around 1 hour. Put on some inspiring music, get moving and have fun.

WEEKS 1–4

The first 4 weeks of the starter plan form a gradual introduction to boxing fitness, emphasizing technique and covering some of the basic punches that you will use throughout your exercise programme. During these first weeks you should stick to Level 1 for all the exercises. By the time you are working week 4 you will be ready to tackle the boxer's circuit (see pages 112–115) on 1 day per week, following the plan below on the other 2 days.

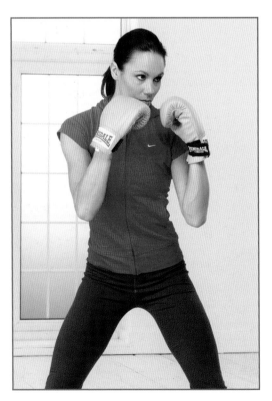

	WEEK 1
WARM-UP	Get moving (see pages 28–29)
	Limber up (see pages 30–31)
	Stretch yourself (see pages 40–41)
CONDITIONING	Get engaged (see page 32)
	Standing posture (see page 36)
	Roll down (see page 38)
	Sideways lean (see page 38)
	Jogging (see page 43)
TECHNIQUE PRACTICE	Forward stance (see page 22)
	Jab (see pages 54–55)
	Cross (see pages 56–57)
COMBINATIONS	Ali shuffle (see page 76)
COOL DOWN	Cool body, cool mind (see pages 48–49)
	Stretch out (see pages 50–51)

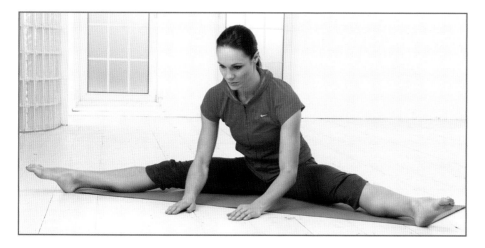

WEEK 2	WEEK 3	WEEK 4
Get moving (see pages 28–29)	Get moving (see pages 28–29)	Get moving (see pages 28–29)
Limber up (see pages 30–31)	Limber up (see pages 30–31)	Limber up (see pages 30–31)
Stretch yourself (see pages 40–41)	Stretch yourself (see pages 40–41)	Stretch yourself (see pages 40–41)
Get engaged (see page 32)	Get engaged (see page 32)	Get engaged (see page 32)
Abs cycling (see pages 34–35)	Abs cycling (see pages 34–35)	Abs cycling (see pages 34–35)
Roll down (see page 38)	Sideways lean (see page 38)	Roll down (see page 38)
Standing posture (see page 36)	Standing posture (see page 36)	Standing posture (see page 36)
Superman (see page 37)	Crunches variation (see page 43)	Back extensions (see page 37)
Crunches (see page 43)	Lunge jumps (see page 104)	Flat bench flies (see page 42)
Push-ups (see page 44)		Skipping (see pages 46–47)
Combat stance (see page 23)	Boxer's guard (see page 20)	Target zones (see page 21)
Jab (see pages 54–55)	Jab (see pages 54–55)	Jab and cross combo (see pages 54–57)
Cross (see pages 56–57)	Cross (see pages 56–57)	Uppercut (see pages 60–61)
Front kick (see pages 78–79)	Hook (see pages 58–59)	Hook (see pages 58–59)
	Uppercut (see pages 60–61)	Back kick (see pages 86–87)
	Side kick (see pages 80–81)	
Spotty dogs (see page 103)	Skipping with rope (see page 47)	Skipping with rope (see page 47)
Cool body, cool mind (see pages 48–49)	Cool body, cool mind (see pages 48–49)	Cool body, cool mind (see pages 48–49)
Stretch out (see pages 50–51)	Stretch out (see pages 50–51)	Stretch out (see pages 50–51)

WEEKS 5–8

During these 4 weeks you will really start to build your fighting repertoire. Here you will begin to work on most of the major punches and kicks, with plenty of time to practise the technique for each one. A variety of more challenging conditioning work and combinations will also get you thinking – and moving. You should now be able to have a go at Level 2 for each exercise, perhaps working up to Level 3 for those you are beginning to find easy. By week 8 you can tackle the pyramid plans (see pages 116–121) on 1 day per week, following the plan below on the other 2 days.

	WEEK 5
WARM-UP	Get moving (see pages 28–29) Limber up (see pages 30–31) Get fired up (see page 19)
CONDITIONING	Get engaged (see page 32) Abs cycling (see pages 34–35) Sideways lean (see page 38) Push-ups (see page 44)
TECHNIQUE PRACTICE	Jab (see pages 54–55) Cross (see pages 56–57) Hook (see pages 58–59) Duck and dive (see page 64) Stacked punch (see pages 66–67) Back kick (see pages 86–87) Jumping back kick (see pages 90–91)
COMBINATIONS	Speedball (see pages 62–63) Ribcage jive (see pages 64–65)
COOL DOWN	Cool body, cool mind (see pages 48–49) Stretch out (see pages 50–51)

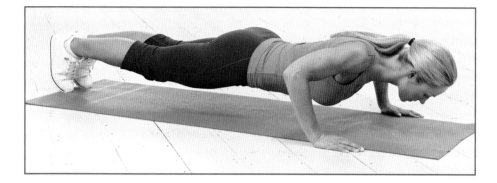

WEEK 6	WEEK 7	WEEK 8
Get moving (see pages 28–29)	Get moving (see pages 28–29)	Get moving (see pages 28–29)
Limber up (see pages 30–31)	Limber up (see pages 30–31)	Limber up (see pages 30–31)
Get fired up (see page 19)	Get fired up (see page 19)	Get fired up (see page 19)
Get engaged (see page 32)	Get engaged (see page 32)	Abs cycling (see pages 34–35)
Abs cycling (see pages 34–35)	Abs cycling variation (see page 35)	Punching abs (see page 33)
Roll down (see page 38)	Sideways lean (see page 38)	Backward bend (see page 39)
Jogging (see page 43)	Backward bend (see page 39)	Crunches variation (see page 43)
	Crunches (see page 43)	
Jab (see pages 54–55)	Hook (see pages 58–59)	Uppercut (see pages 60–61)
Cross (see pages 56–57)	Duck and dive (see page 64)	Duck and dive (see page 64)
Hook (see pages 58–59)	Stacked punch (see pages 66–67)	Stacked punch (see pages 66–67)
Duck and dive (see page 64)	Throw and catch (see page 74)	Front kick (see pages 78–79)
Stacked punch (see pages 66–67)	Front kick (see pages 78–79)	Side kick (see pages 80–81)
Throw and catch (see page 74)	Side kick (see pages 80–81)	Spinning side kick (see pages
Front kick (see pages 78–79)	Roundhouse kick (see pages 84–85)	82–83)
Speedball (see pages 62–63)	Speedball (see pages 62–63)	Speedball (see pages 62–63)
Twist it further (see page 65)	Boxer's adage (see page 73)	Yoga hold (see page 72)
		Ali shuffle (see page 76)
Cool body, cool mind (see pages 48–49)	Cool body, cool mind (see pages 48–49)	Cool body, cool mind (see pages 48–49)
Stretch out (see pages 50–51)	Stretch out (see pages 50–51)	Stretch out (see pages 50–51)

WEEKS 9–12

These final 4 weeks complete your full repertoire of kicks and punches. You will also increase your practice of conditioning and combination work, adding even more moves to make sure you are fit enough – because by week 12 you will be performing all the punches and kicks you have learned in this book, so you'd better be ready for it! You should be working comfortably at Level 2 for all exercises, while Level 3 will become progressively easier.

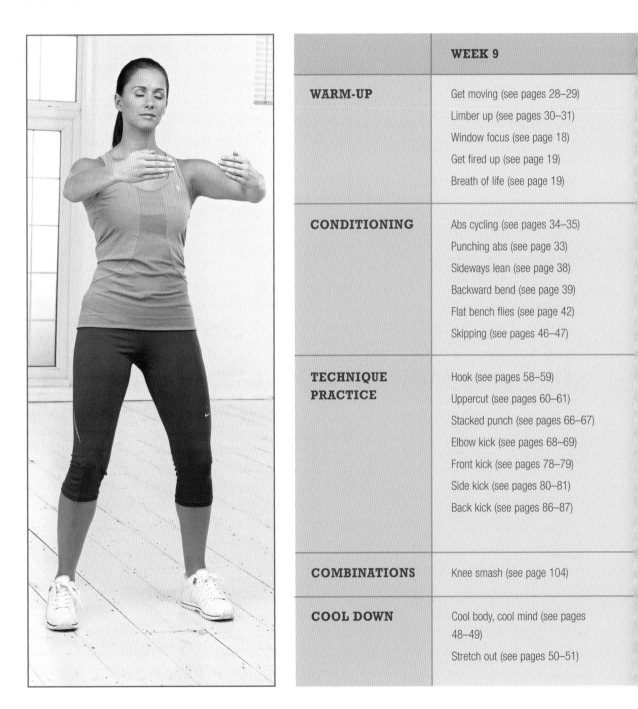

	WEEK 9
WARM-UP	Get moving (see pages 28–29)
	Limber up (see pages 30–31)
	Window focus (see page 18)
	Get fired up (see page 19)
	Breath of life (see page 19)
CONDITIONING	Abs cycling (see pages 34–35)
	Punching abs (see page 33)
	Sideways lean (see page 38)
	Backward bend (see page 39)
	Flat bench flies (see page 42)
	Skipping (see pages 46–47)
TECHNIQUE PRACTICE	Hook (see pages 58–59)
	Uppercut (see pages 60–61)
	Stacked punch (see pages 66–67)
	Elbow kick (see pages 68–69)
	Front kick (see pages 78–79)
	Side kick (see pages 80–81)
	Back kick (see pages 86–87)
COMBINATIONS	Knee smash (see page 104)
COOL DOWN	Cool body, cool mind (see pages 48–49)
	Stretch out (see pages 50–51)

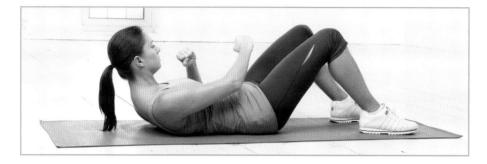

WEEK 10	WEEK 11	WEEK 12
Get moving (see pages 28–29)	Get moving (see pages 28–29)	Get moving (see pages 28–29)
Limber up (see pages 30–31)	Limber up (see pages 30–31)	Limber up (see pages 30–31)
Window focus (see page 18)	Window focus (see page 18)	Window focus (see page 18)
Get fired up (see page 19)	Get fired up (see page 19)	Get fired up (see page 19)
Breath of life (see page 19)	Breath of life (see page 19)	Breath of life (see page 19)
Abs cycling (see pages 34–35)	Abs cycling (see pages 34–35)	Abs cycling (see pages 34–35)
Punching abs (see page 33)	Punching abs (see page 33)	Punching abs (see page 33)
Backward bend (see page 39)	Backward bend (see page 39)	Backward bend (see page 39)
Push-ups variation 1 (see page 45)	Push-ups variation 1 (see page 45)	Push-ups variation 1 (see page 45)
Skipping (see pages 46–47)	Skipping (see pages 46–47)	Skipping (see pages 46–47)
Jab (see pages 54–55)	Jab (see pages 54–55)	All punches and kicks (see pages 54–69 and 78–91)
Cross (see pages 56–57)	Cross (see pages 56–57)	
Hook (see pages 58–59)	Hook (see pages 58–59)	
Uppercut (see pages 60–61)	Uppercut (see pages 60–61)	
Elbow kick variation (see page 69)	Side kick (see pages 80–81)	
Front kick (see pages 78–79)	Roundhouse kick (see pages 84–85)	
Side kick (see pages 80–81)	Back kick variation (see page 87)	
Roundhouse kick (see pages 84–85)	Jump kick (see pages 88–89)	
Speedball (see pages 62–63)	Gallop with twist (see page 105)	Sumo squat (see page 75)
Cool body, cool mind (see pages 48–49)	Cool body, cool mind (see pages 48–49)	Cool body, cool mind (see pages 48–49)
Stretch out (see pages 50–51)	Stretch out (see pages 50–51)	Stretch out (see pages 50–51)

footwork FRENZY

Try this for an agility workout. Here you will combine a variety of punches and kicks with some fancy footwork. Changing direction and the way you are facing throughout the workout will rapidly bring your mobility and focus up to a new level.

WARM-UP
Skipping – 10 minutes (see pages 46–47).

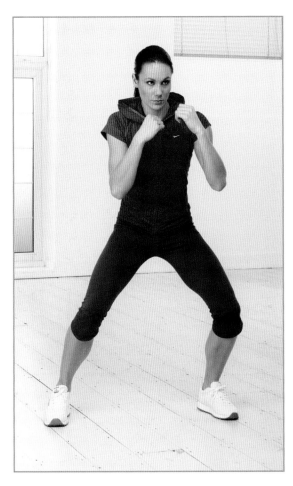

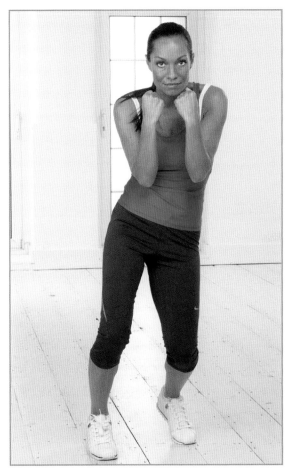

GALLOP
Start with small sideways steps from one side of your space to the other (see page 77). Repeat 4–5 times.

ALI SHUFFLE
Now add some Ali shuffles (see page 76). Keep your TVA engaged and fists lifted as you bounce lightly from foot to foot on the spot. You can turn and face whichever way you need to as the Ali shuffle moves you around your space. Keep going for 1 minute.

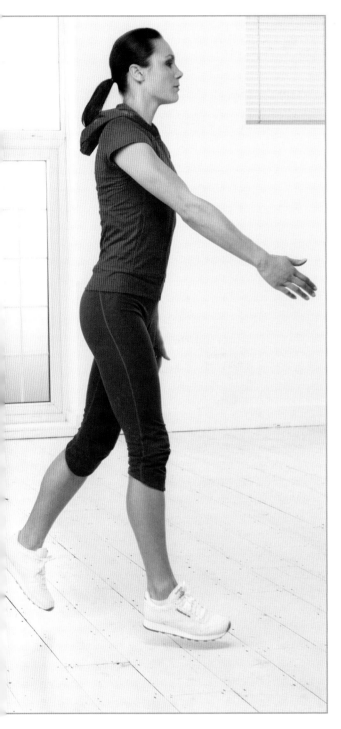

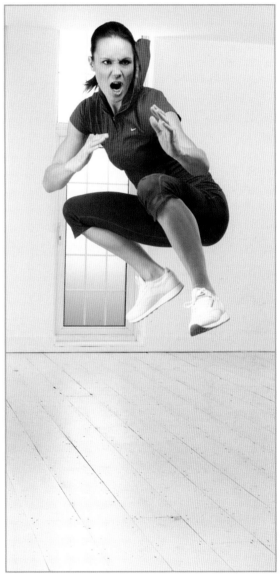

SPOTTY DOGS

This is a classic aerobic move that can be used by martial artists as well as boxers. Bounce your weight from one foot to the other, first with one foot in front of the other. Now swap your feet forward and back as you bounce. Your arms should move forward and back as well. Keep going for 1 minute.

STANCE JUMP

From spotty dogs, go back into the Ali shuffle and then jump with both feet into a wide squat. Repeat once more.

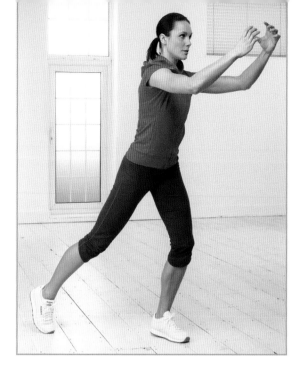
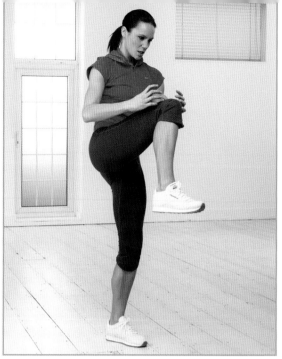

KNEE SMASH

1 Now add some knee lifts. Keep your body lifted and lift your arms above your head.

2 Now lift your knee up towards your chest, bringing your arms down as you do so. Add in a hop as you change legs, lifting your knee and bringing your arms down with aggression. Repeat 5 times on each knee.

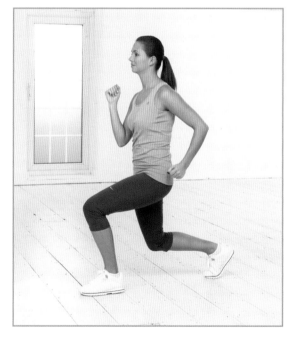
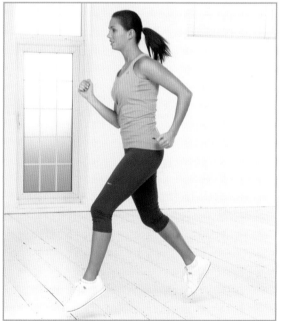

LUNGE JUMPS

1 Now add some higher impact moves. From the Ali shuffle, jump into a lunge position with one leg forward and the knee bent.

2 Jump straight up to change legs and land in a lunge with the other leg in front. Repeat the jump to swap legs 4 times.

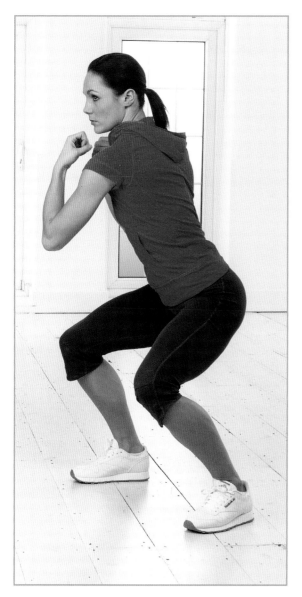

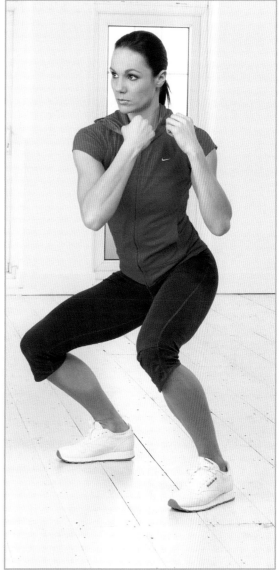

GALLOP WITH TWIST

1 Finally, come back to the side-to-side gallop, and as you reach the edge of your space stay in the gallop on the spot as you twist your ribcage, bringing your elbow to the front as you do so.

2 Now do the same with the other elbow. Really twist and turn your upper body to move your arms as you bring first one elbow to the front and then the other. Repeat the gallop with twist once in each direction.

COOL-DOWN

Stretch out (see pages 50–51).

quick workout: PUNCHES

Put on some upbeat music that lasts for around 5 minutes and then work each move in this routine for a count of 8. Galloping one way across your space counts as 1 repetition. Moving in time to the music should help you to maintain the momentum.

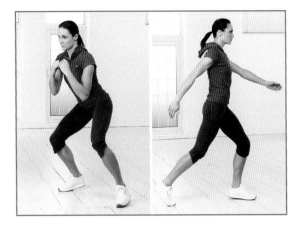

1 Gallop – 4 times, then spotty dogs – 4 times.

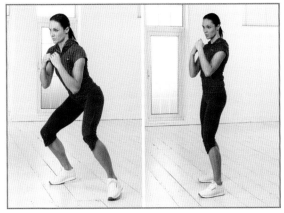

2 Gallop – 4 times, then combat stance and pulse back and forth.

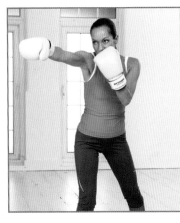

3 Perform 2 jabs with each arm – 4 times.

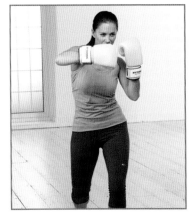

4 Perform 2 hooks with each arm – 4 times.

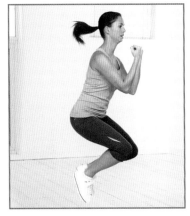

5 Stance jump into forward stance to change position.

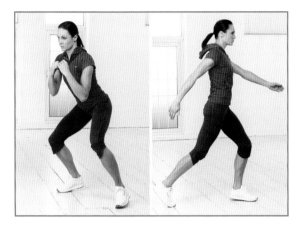

6 Gallop – 4 times, then spotty dogs – 4 times.

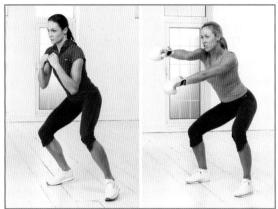

7 Gallop – 4 times, then stacked punch – 4 times.

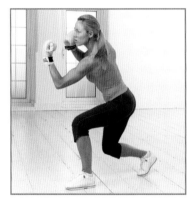

8 Perform 2 uppercuts with each arm – 4 times.

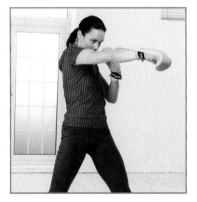

9 Perform 2 cross punches with each arm – 4 times.

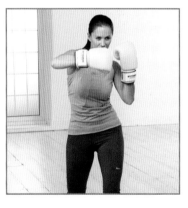

10 Perform 2 hooks with each arm – 4 times.

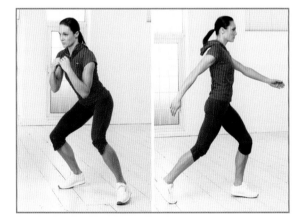

11 Gallop – 4 times, then spotty dogs – 4 times.

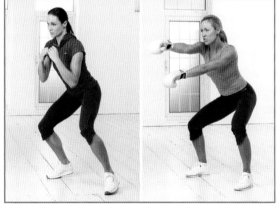

12 Gallop – 4 times, then stacked punch – 4 times.

Repeat the sequence until the music ends.

quick workout: KICKS

Put on some lively music that lasts for 6–8 minutes and then work this routine in counts of 8.

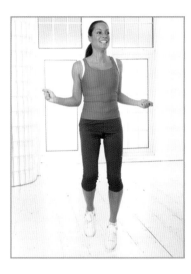

1 Shadow skip – 8 times.

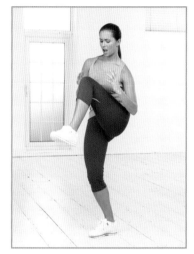

2 Knee smash – 8 times.

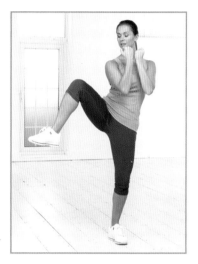

3 Knee lift out to the side – 8 times.

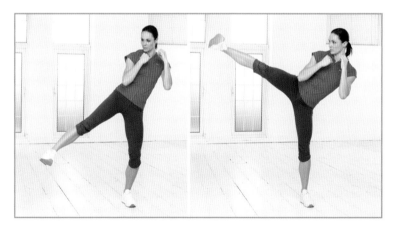

4 Side kick, low, then high – 8 times.

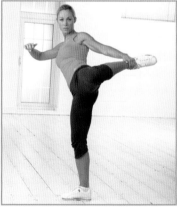

5 Throw and catch – 8 times.

6 Roundhouse kick – 8 times.

7 Thigh stretch – for a count of 8.

8 Shadow skip – 8 times.

9 Jogging – for a count of 8.

10 Shadow skip – 16 times.

11 Front kick – 8 times.

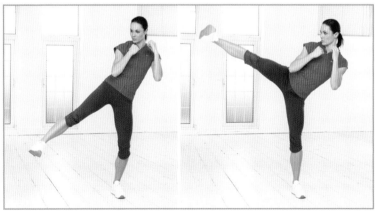

12 Side kick, low, then high – 8 times.

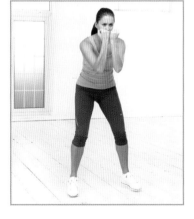

13 Stance jump, then bounce – 8 times.

Repeat the sequence until the music ends.

quick workout: COMBO

Put on some fast music that works in counts of 8, then work this routine to the same timing.
Galloping one way across your space counts as 1 repetition.

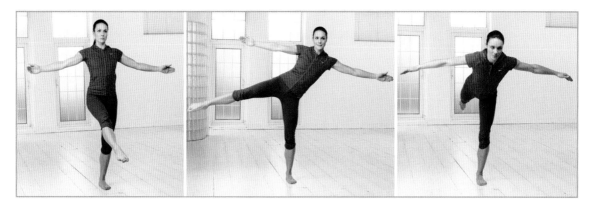

1 Boxer's adage – for a count of 8.

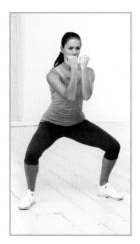 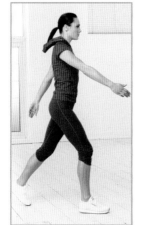 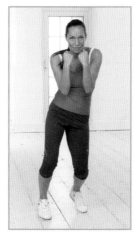 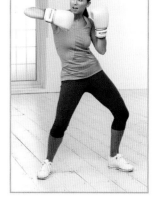

2 Stance jump into a low stance with your feet 1½ hip widths apart, to change position.

3 Spotty dogs – 16 times.

4 Ali shuffle – for a count of 8.

5 Elbow kick to the left, then right – 8 times.

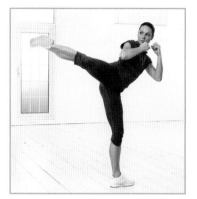

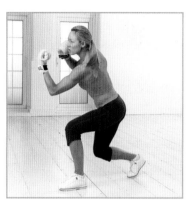

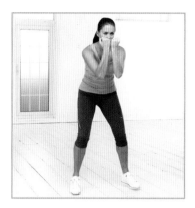

6 Back kick, then get down low and bounce – for a count of 8.

7 Uppercut, low into the body – 4 times.

8 Bounce in forward stance – 8 times.

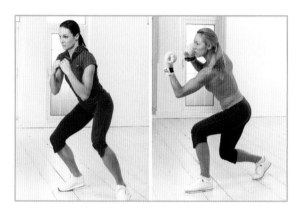

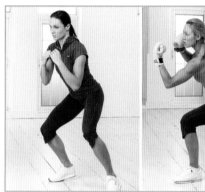

9 Gallop to left, then uppercut – 4 times.

10 Gallop to right, then uppercut – 4 times.

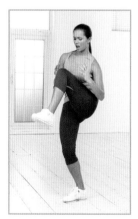

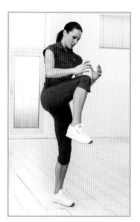

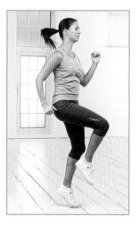

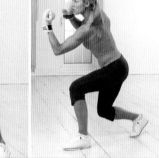

11 Knee smash, softly – 4 times.

12 Knee smash, aggressively – 4 times.

13 Jogging – for a count of 8.

14 Lunge jump to change position.

Repeat from Step 3 (spotty dogs) for as long as you like or until the music ends.

boxer's CIRCUIT

This is a great conditioning workout that incorporates many of the moves and punches you have learned. It is set out like a boxing match, but backwards – so you have 1-minute rounds followed by 3-minute cardiovascular recovery sections. You will need a skipping rope, boxing gloves (if you have them) and a mat. Now put on some thumping music and get going!

WARM-UP

Always prepare your body for the workout by warming up (see pages 28–31).

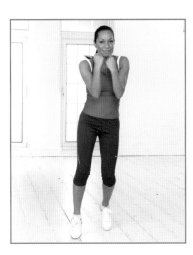

RECOVERY ROUND 1: ALI SHUFFLE (3 MINUTES)

Shuffle on the spot, keeping your fists lifted, adding the occasional duck and dive as you recover.

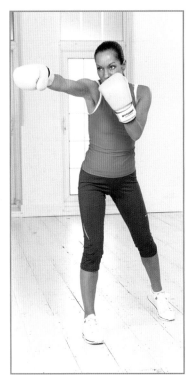

STATION 1 (1 MINUTE)

Jab with both hands for 30 seconds. Remember your technique: hit out in front of you with fists high, arms rebounding, as fast as you can. For the last 30 seconds add some cross punches with your other arm – don't forget to turn your foot as you punch.

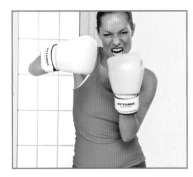

STATION 2 (1 MINUTE)

Start throwing some hooks with each hand. Remember your focus and mindset: remind yourself where you're aiming and throw the punch with aggression.

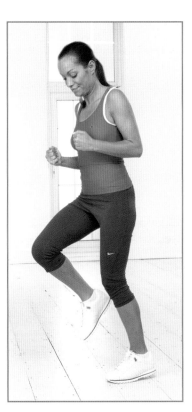

RECOVERY ROUND 2: JOGGING (3 MINUTES)

Jog on the spot to recover. Swing your arms to loosen them, then lift your knees up as high as you can in front of you. Now let them drop a little and jog again, gently at first and then really speed up.

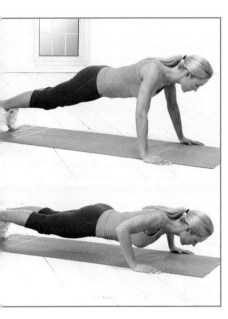

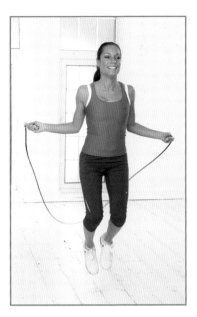

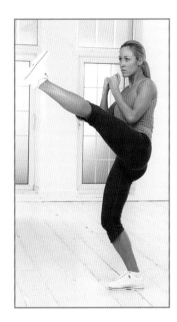

STATION 3 (1 MINUTE)

Get down on your knees and attempt some push-ups. Perform some with your arms wide and some with them narrow. Try to keep going for the whole minute.

RECOVERY ROUND 3: SKIPPING (3 MINUTES)

Get up off the floor and grab your skipping rope. Recover as you swing the rope and keep the skipping going. If the rope catches, just untangle and carry on.

STATION 5 (1 MINUTE)

Try some front kicks. Set your stance, move about and then unleash the kicks. Do enough on each leg to keep going for a minute.

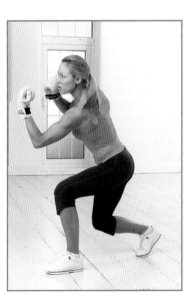

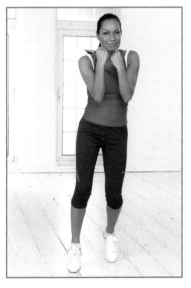

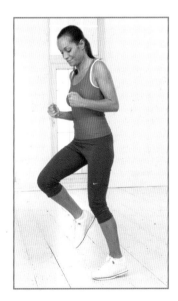

STATION 4 (1 MINUTE)

Perform uppercuts with your right and left arms. Vary the speed and the focal point. Hit some high at your imaginary opponent's chin and others lower, at the solar plexus.

RECOVERY ROUND 4: ALI SHUFFLE (3 MINUTES)

As round 1.

RECOVERY ROUND 5: JOGGING (3 MINUTES)

As round 2.

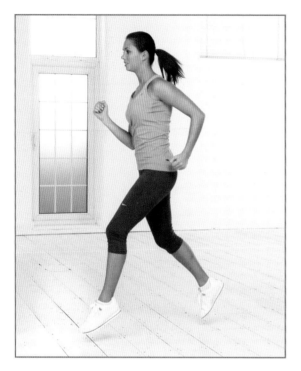

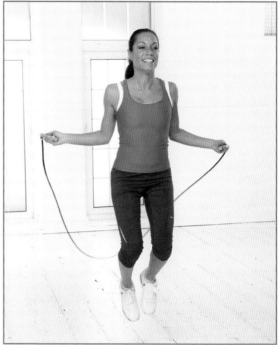

STATION 6 (1 MINUTE)

Now up the pace by doing some lunge jumps. Set up the lunge, then spring into the air and land with your other foot in front. Try to complete as many as you can in a minute.

RECOVERY ROUND 6: SKIPPING
(3 MINUTES)

As round 3.

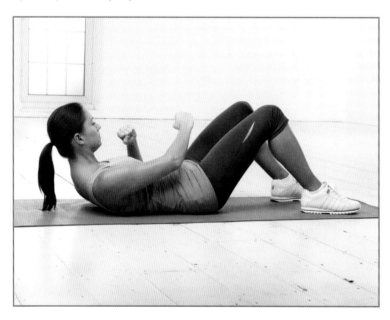

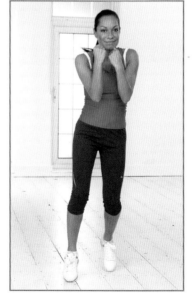

STATION 7 (1 MINUTE)

Hit the floor to do some punching abs. Lie on your back with your knees bent, then curl your head and shoulders off the floor, as you punch forward as many times as you can in a minute.

RECOVERY ROUND 7: ALI SHUFFLE (3 MINUTES)

As round 1.

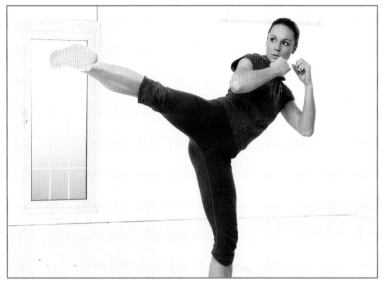

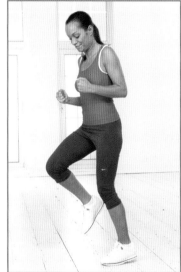

STATION 8 (1 MINUTE)

Throw some back kicks behind you to surprise your opponent.
Try to back kick to every side of your space as you spin and kick,
and keep going for a full minute.

RECOVERY ROUND 8: JOGGING (3 MINUTES)

As round 2.

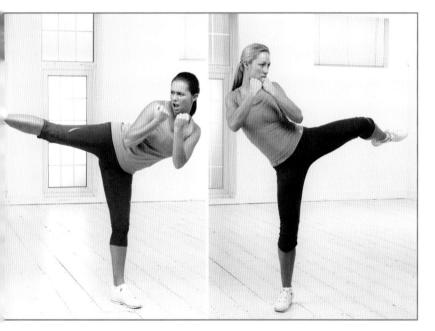

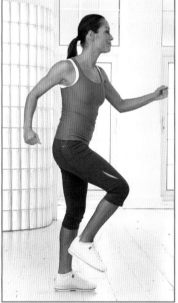

STATION 9 (1 MINUTE)

Alternate some side kicks with roundhouse kicks to remind
yourself of the difference. Kick to each side of your space, and
try kicking higher and lower.

COOL-DOWN

Start by jogging on the spot, then slow
down to recover slightly. Now march
on the spot, swinging your arms and
breathing deeply. Give yourself a towel
down and a pat on the back for a
workout well done!

the PYRAMID PRINCIPLE

This is a great way to put a fun workout together. It involves building up blocks of an exercise, doing just 10 repetitions each time before moving on. Restricting the number of repetitions means you can perform each one perfectly without any loss of form, yet as the blocks build up you will really feel the intensity of this regime. The pyramid training principle was originally used for boxers in the gym and has now passed into the fitness world as a great alternative to the circuit.

REMEMBER...

✳ Each exercise is only performed 10 times before moving on to the next block.

✳ Each time you hit the edge of the pyramid, you perform the exercise interval for 1 minute and then return to the start of the blocks that remain.

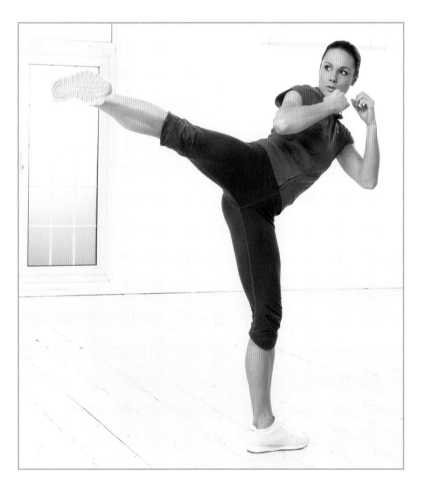

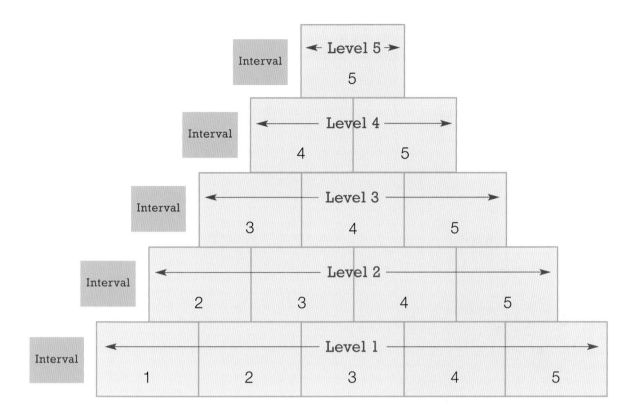

PYRAMID RULES

Study the chart above and then follow the instructions below. It may help to cross off each square as you complete it, so that you can chart where you are.

1 Perform 10 reps from Level 1. Go to the exercise interval.

2 Start on Level 1 again and perform 10 reps from here, then move up a level and perform 10 repetitions from Level 2. Go to the exercise interval.

3 Start on Level 1 again and perform 10 reps, then move up to Level 2 and perform 10 reps, and then to Level 3 and perform 10 reps. Go to the exercise interval.

4 Carry on all the way up the pyramid in the same way, starting at Level 1 each time, until you reach the top.

5 Now start from Level 5 and do all the exercises coming down the pyramid. Go to the exercise interval.

6 Go back up to Level 4 (you have finished with Level 5) and again do all the exercises coming down.

7 Carry on working your way down in this way until you have completed Level 1. Finish with a cool down interval, such as marching on the spot – you are done!

Once you have understood how the pyramid works, you can make up your own versions using all the different moves and strikes you have learned in any combination that suits. To start you off, two different types of pyramid are provided on the following pages.

combination PYRAMID

This pyramid is designed to combine a number of the moves you have learned. Put on some loud background music, but take your time with each repetition and perform a full minute of the exercise interval each time you reach the edge of the pyramid.

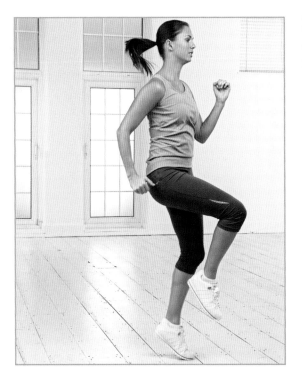

EXERCISE INTERVAL

Jog on the spot or Ali shuffle while you pound that speedball over and over. This interval lasts for 1 minute.

LEVEL 1

Side kick with jab and cross Fix your sights on an imaginary opponent at your side. Gallop in to side kick them, then follow this by throwing them a jab and a cross punch.

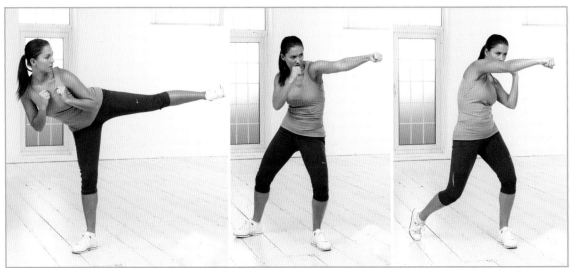

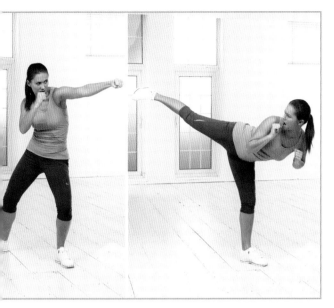

LEVEL 2

Jab, jab, back kick Start with your left foot and fist in front. Step forward with each jab of your left hand, then surprise the opponent coming at you from behind with a back kick. Alternate with the other side leading.

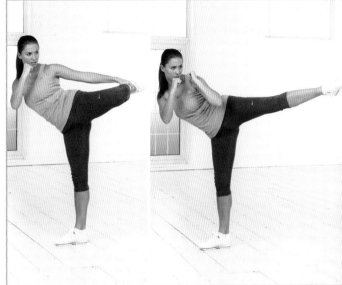

LEVEL 3

Throw and catch, roundhouse Throw and catch your left leg, then throw and extend for the roundhouse kick. Alternate legs during your 10 repetitions.

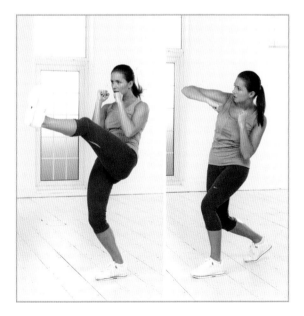

LEVEL 4

Jump kick and elbow Swing into the jump kick and finish with a decisive elbow to the side.

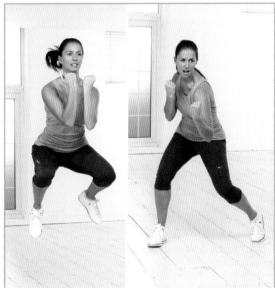

LEVEL 5

Jump squat with 10 uppercuts Finish the top level with a jump that lands you in a wide squat. Bend your legs low and then pummel your opponent with 10 uppercuts in quick succession.

CV pyramid

This cardiovascular pyramid demonstrates just how flexible this method of working out can be, and how you can exercise your heart and lungs as well as your arms, legs and abdominals as you burn fat *and* tone your body! This is a tough pyramid, so you may want to practise by doing just the 'up' phase to begin with. As you get fitter, you can add the 'down' phase.

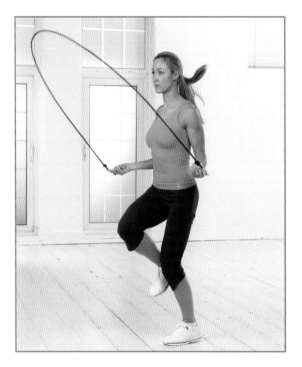

EXERCISE INTERVAL

Grab the skipping rope and try to keep the boxer's bounce going for 1 minute.

LEVEL 1

Gallop left, 3 jabs, 3 crosses; gallop right, 3 jabs, 3 crosses
Gallop to your left across your space as far as you can, then throw 6 jabs and crosses before speeding over to the other side and repeating the punches. This forms 1 complete repetition.

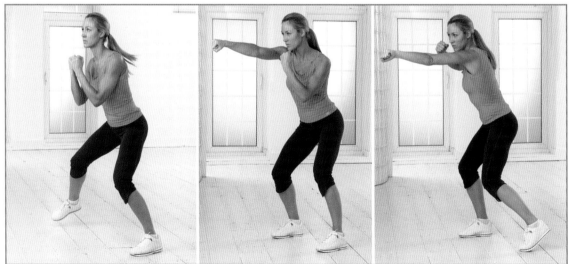

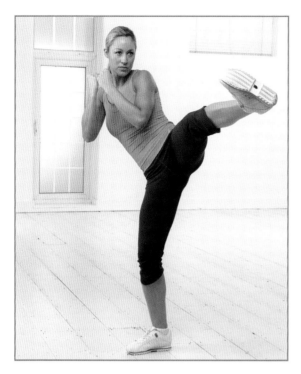

LEVEL 2

Side kicks Side kick fast and hard, first to your imaginary opponent's ankle, then higher to the waist, using alternate legs. Each low and high kick forms 1 repetition.

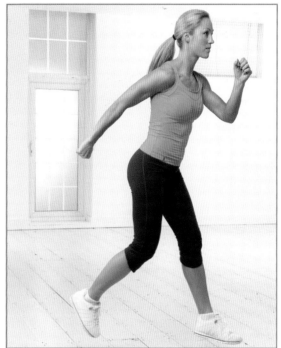

LEVEL 3

Spotty dogs Jump your left leg and arm in front, then bounce your right leg and arm forward. Each right and left forms 1 repetition.

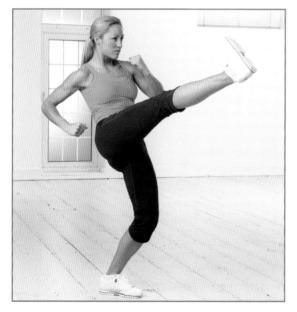

LEVEL 4

Front kicks Perform 10 front kicks with all the power of an expert martial artist, alternating your legs.

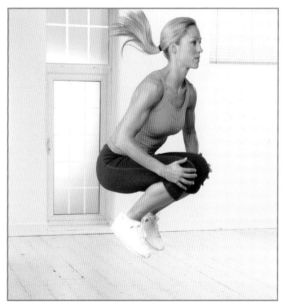

LEVEL 5

Tuck jumps Stand with your feet hip width apart, bend your knees and spring up into the air. Try to bring your knees up to your chest as you jump and land softly by bending your knees.

de-stress YOURSELF

By now you will have realized how a good kick-and-punch routine can get virtually every muscle in your body working. However, it is always important to relax your body and mind after you have worked out. This doesn't need to be done directly after you have finished exercising – you may wish to perform some of the stretches on pages 50–51 first – but carrying out relaxation work at some point will really boost your physical and mental well-being.

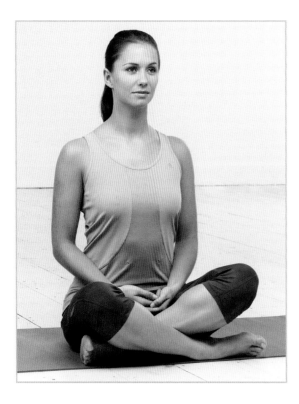

2 Try to allow your mind to settle. Focus on your breathing: observe and listen to the sound of your body taking in air. Try to think of nothing in particular – which will probably mean everything at once! Your aim is simply to become an observer of your own mind. Watch the thoughts and feelings that come into your mind as you remain quite still, but try not to follow any of them. Try not to think about the workout you have just done, or your plans for tomorrow – just observe your thoughts.

3 Keep breathing regularly and naturally as you watch your thoughts skit across your brain, like stars streaking across the night sky. Each time your mind wanders and pulls you off with a particular thought, try to return to your breathing and prevent further activity! This kind of work takes practice but reaps many benefits.

4 As you develop the skill of controlling your mind, you will be able to focus better as you practise your moves and relax more afterwards. Practise this mind relaxation for just 5 minutes to start with, and if you enjoy it you can build up to longer sessions of body and mind relaxation.

RELEASE YOUR MIND

1 Sit or lie in a comfortable position, but not one in which you are likely to fall asleep! Meditation is definitely not about sleeping. You don't need to be still in your body in order to still your mind, but when you first begin learning these skills it's easier if mind and body work together, so keep still through your meditation.

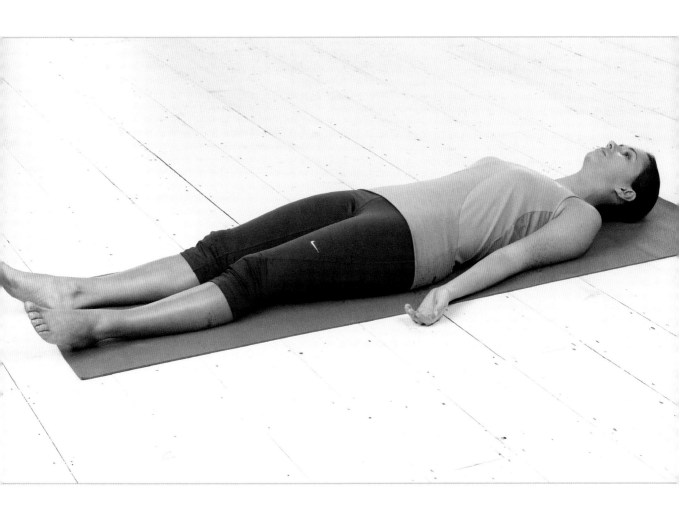

RELEASE YOUR BODY

1 Lie flat on the floor, preferably on your back or in a similar comfortable position, in a warm room. Simply rest for a few seconds in this position to allow your body to settle.

2 Now start at the lower end of your body and scrunch up your toes, squeezing them tight, then release the tension and allow them to relax completely.

3 Point your toes to tense your calf muscles strongly, then release the squeeze and notice how your muscles relax into the floor.

4 Without tensing your lower legs, tighten the muscles on the front of your thighs, pulling up your knee caps, then release. Feel the front of your thighs relax and imagine that relaxation extending around to the back of them as well.

5 Squeeze your buttocks strongly and contract your abdominals by pushing your lower back into the floor. Release both sets of muscles and feel your torso sink to the floor.

6 Contract your shoulders upwards towards your ears and at the same time squeeze your hands into fists and press them hard against the floor. Now release the tension and feel the whole of your arms relaxing on to the floor.

7 Finally, press your head into the floor and press your shoulders down towards your ribcage. Now release this tension and feel your neck and face relaxing. Take several more minutes to let each of these changes register, working back through your body and noticing how each part is now relaxed and falling more heavily into the floor as the muscles let go. Slowly bring awareness back to your abdominals and take a really deep breath to stimulate you out of your relaxation.

INDEX

ACKNOWLEDEMENTS

Hamlyn would like to thank the following for supplying props for photography:
Physical Company
2a Desborough Industrial Park
Desborough Park Road
High Wycombe
Buckinghamshire
HP12 3BG
www.physicalcompany.co.uk

Powerhouse Fitness
129 St. John's Hill
Battersea
London
SW11 1TD
www.powerhouse-fitness.co.uk

Executive Editor Jane McIntosh
Senior Editor Charlotte Macey
Executive Art Editor Sally Bond
Designer Janis Utton
Production Controller Carolin Stransky

Photography Mike Prior
Make-up Andrew Savage

Special photography
©Octopus Publishing Group Limited/Mike Prior